Chén Xiūyuán's 陳修園

金匱方歌括

Formulas from the Golden Cabinet with Songs

Jīn Guì Fāng Gē Kuò

Volumes IV - VI

Eran Even Dr. TCM, R.Ac.

The Chinese Medicine Database
www.cm-db.com
Portland, Oregon

Formulas from the Golden Cabinet with Songs

金匱方歌括

Jīn Guì Fāng Gē Kuò

Volumes IV - VI

Eran Even

1017 SW Morrison #306
Portland, OR 97205 USA

COMP designation original Chinese work and English translation

Cover Design by Jonathan Schell L.Ac.
Library of Congress Cataloging-in-Publication Data:

Chen, Xiuyuan, 1753-1823.
[Formulas from the Golden Cabinet with Songs. English]
Jin Gui Fang Ge Kuo = Formulas from the Golden Cabinet with Songs IV-VI
/ translation Eran Even
p. cm.
Includes Index.
ISBN 978-0-9799552-8-0 (alk. paper)
Medicine, Chinese I. Even, Eran. II. Title: Formulas from the Golden Cabinet with Songs
III. Title: Vol. IV - VI

International Standard Book Number (ISBN): 978-0-9799552-8-0
Printed in the United States of America

Contents

Contents

Chén Xiūyuán has quite a large reputation in China, as one of the brightest and most famous doctors of the last 250 years. Even though he did not practice medicine as his career but served as a senior government official in many regions, medicine was his true love.

A friend offered this depiction of him.

> My old friend Chén Xiūyuán was very skilled in the methods of Qí Bó and Huáng Dì (Chinese medicine). He was very self-confident and considered himself the reincarnation of the Chángshā master (Zhāng Zhòngjǐng), which caused many physicians to tease him. Once there was a critically ill patient whose condition was so severe no physician could help, so Chén went to visit the patient. On arrival he took off his hat, laid it on the table, and stretched out his hand to feel the patient's pulse. He looked up with his eyes glinting, and after quite some time, laughed and said, "This is not an uncommon disease, it's just that [the previous] doctor interfered and made it worse." The patient's family said, "But he's a very famous doctor!" Chén abruptly said "It's wrong!" The patient's family said that this particular doctor modeled himself after Zhū Dānxī, Zhāng Jǐngyuè, Wáng Kěntāng, and Lǐ Gǎo, to which Chén responded "Then it's more wrong! Can these physicians cure any disease?" He prescribed a formula while continuing to scold [the family]. When he finished, he began to discuss and admire his prescription, stood up to weigh out the ingredients, and cooked them himself. He urged the patient to drink the decoction, and the results turned out exactly as he said.[1]

Chén Xiūyuán is highly respected and beloved. He is respected for his perseverance, his self-confidence, and his ability to clearly differentiate what he liked, and what he detested. He was a very opinionated doctor who had very strong resentment against the doctors of his time who neglected the classics and revered the medical style of the *Jīn, Yuán,* and *Míng* doctors. From his viewpoint, the real medical sage was the *Hàn* Dynasties' Zhāng Zhòngjǐng. He believed that all doctors must read the *Shāng Hán Lùn,* and the *Jīn Guì Yào Lüè,* and in his own clinical practice, he mainly used classical formulas. Chén Xiūyuán adhered to tradition, emphasizing the importance of the classics while being mindful to follow the rules of Chinese medicine. He is a true representative of the Chinese medicine *Jīng Fāng* current. *Jīng Fāng* is the abbreviation for formulas from the classics, and is also short for the experienced formulas of the classical periods. The formulas recorded in Zhāng Zhòngjǐng's *Shāng Hán Lùn* and *Jīn Guì Yào Lüè* are the "classical formulas." *Jīng Fāng* is canonical and highly effective, thus it is the standard for clinical practice and the academic foundation of

1. Taken from Jiǎng Qìnglíng's preface to Chén Xiūyuán's *Shén Nóng Běn Cǎo Jīng Dú*《神農本草經讀》(Reading the Divine Farmer's Classic of Materia Medica).

Chinese medicine. Chén Xiūyuán devoted his entire life to studying the work of Zhāng Zhòngjǐng and spreading *Jīng Fāng*. In his lifetime he wrote numerous and highly accessible medical books, including the *Jīn Guì Yào Lüè Qiǎn Zhù* 《 金匮要略浅注 》(Shallow Commentary on the *Jīn Guì Yào Lüè*), *Shāng Hán Lùn Qiǎn Zhù* 《 傷寒論淺注 》(Shallow Commentary on the *Shāng Hán Lùn*), *Cháng Shā Fāng Gē Kuò* 《 長沙方歌括 》(Formulas with Songs from Chàng Shā), and the *Yī Xué Sān Zì Jīng* 《 醫學三字經 》(Three Character Classic on Medical Studies). Most of these books are very popular and widely circulated, and have been published repeatedly.

However, as far as I am aware, the *Jīn Guì Fāng Gē Kuò* is (Chén's) first work translated into English. This book is Chén Xiūyuán's primary compilation, for which his children provided assistance in composing the work. The book contains various songs or poems used to aid in the ease of memorizing the various compositions, functions, main indications, medicinal dosages, and cooking methods of the formulas found within the *Jīn Guì Yào Lüè*. Following the songs, each one of Zhāng Zhòngjǐng's formulas is accompanied by a brief commentary in order to assist the reader in understanding the significance and usage of these classical formulas. The publishing of Eran's translation of Chén Xiūyuán's *Jīn Guì Fāng Gē Kuò* into English is something that should please many. Of course having more of Chén Xiūyuán's work, as well as other ancient *Jīng Fāng* contemporaries' works, translated into English would also be very welcome indeed!

In recent years the reputation of *Jīng Fāng* has grown considerably, as many Chinese medicine colleagues and friends overseas are beginning to study and apply these classical formulas. This indicates that the second wave of the worldwide enthusiasm for Chinese medicine is coming. It can be said that the first wave began in the 1970s with acupuncture as the vehicle, while the second wave is currently brewing, characterized by the application of Chinese medicinals, for which *Jīng Fāng* is the vehicle. I usually say that there are two treasures in Chinese medicine, one being acupuncture, and the other *Jīng Fāng*. Acupuncture is very convenient to carry around in order to be used for first aid treatments, while *Jīng Fāng* is schematic and deliberate, which is very good for regulation and standardization. While they both originate from Chinese traditional medical techniques of ancient times, they are universal as well because they are the crystallization of human intelligence. Eran's translation of the *Jīn Guì Fāng Gè Kuō* is a very significant work in the internationalization of Chinese medical studies.

It is my sincere hope that readers enjoy Eran's translation of the *Jīn Guì Fāng Gē Kuò*, and that they enjoy the work of Chén Xiūyuán, classic formulas, and Chinese medicinals!

Professor Huáng Huáng (黄煌)
Nán Jīng University of Chinese Medicine
May 27, 2014

Foreword by Z'ev Rosenberg, L.Ac.

Jīn Guì Fāng Gē Kuò《金匱方歌括》(Formulas from the Golden Cabinet with Songs), Volumes IV-VI, completes this work of Chén Xiūyuán 陳修園, a commentary on the *Jīn Guì Yào Lüè* (Prescriptions from the Golden Cabinet). So what is the value of reading commentaries on classical medical texts?

While the originals of *Shāng Hán Lùn* and *Jīn Guì Yào Lüè* are at first glance relatively simple in writing style and delivery, there is a great deal of complexity just beneath the surface. Zhāng Zhòngjǐng studied and compiled a great deal of source material, including the *Sù Wèn, Líng Shū,* and *Tāng Yè Jīng* (Decoction Classic) to produce his work.

Sophisticated applications of five-phase theory, combinations of medicinals in formulas, channel theory from the *Sù Wèn,* and pulse diagnostics are just some of the threads that brought the *Shāng Hán Zá Bìng Lùn* together as a coherent text (before being recompiled by Wáng Shūhē into two texts, the *Shāng Hán Lùn* and *Jīn Guì Yào Lüè*). The purpose of Chén Xiūyuán's work was to bring a depth of inquiry to the material, to reveal what is underneath the surface, and to open the garden of the text through a lyrical style ("songs") that facilitates easy learning and memorization. It often adds the clinical experience of the commentator as well, offering a historical perspective on practice in later eras (after the *Hàn* Dynasty, when these texts were written). Dr. Chén was one of the foremost *Qīng* Dynasty scholars of classical medicine, and in his translation, Eran Even gives us a rare glimpse into the thinking mode and practice of a great physician.

When practicing Chinese herbal medicine, it is not enough to match biomedical diseases or simple *zàng-fǔ* patterns to formulas, or treat symptomatically. We must understand the underlying *bìng jī* 病機 (pathomechanisms) at work if we wish to have any hope of clinical success. Commentators such as Chén Xiūyuán "open up" the original text and the formulas, allowing us to understand the synergism of the ingredients chosen according to very specific rules, and how by resolving these pathomechanisms classical formulas can treat a wide range of illnesses and clinical patterns. The key principle here is *qì huà* 氣化 (qì transformation), understanding the normal movement of qì and blood as they ascend and descend through the sānjiāo (three burners). Classical formulas seek to rectify qì transformation so that the body and mind can effectively eliminate disease factors on its own, rather than suppressing bodily or mental and emotional functions to do so.

"Even" in Hebrew means a stone or rock, personifying solidity and stability. Eran Even is a young man who has made great strides in his Chinese medical scholarship, having produced a blog (http://chinesemedicinecases.com) that contains translations of case histories of great physicians, such as Féng Shìlún, Huáng Huáng, Liú Dùzhōu, Hú Xīshù, and many others who have focused on the *Shāng Hán Lùn* and *Jīn Guì* as the primary source texts for their practices. Translating texts such as the *Jīn Guì Fāng Gē Kuò* is difficult at best, and Eran has done a marvelous job in rendering the original *Qīng* Dynasty Chinese into English. This translation is an important achievement that deserves wide study.

Z'ev Rosenberg, L.Ac.
Chair emeritus, Pacific College of Oriental Medicine, San Diego
Professor, Alembic and Xinglin Institutes, San Diego

With this edition of the *Jīn Guì Fāng Gē Kuò* Volumes IV-VI we have followed the same conversions for weight and measures as with the *Jīn Guì Fāng Gē Kuò* Volumes I-III. For convenience, we have added these tables into this book as well.

Volume:

5 dǒu	斗	=	1 hú	斛	=	10 liters
10 shēng	升	=	1 dǒu	斗	=	2 liters
10 gě	合	=	1 shēng	升	=	200ml
			1 gě	合	=	20ml

Weight:

1 jīn	斤	48g
1 liǎng	兩	3g
1 qián	錢	0.3g
1 fēn	分	0.75g

We believe that presenting the dosage in grams and milliliters will save the practitioner time when adopting these valuable formulas in your clinical practice.

Jonathan Schell L.Ac.
The Chinese Medicine Database
Portland, OR
September, 4, 2014

Translator's Preface and Acknowledgments

The translator is not a ferryman for the meaning of the words, but the author of their web of new relations. And he is not the painter of the light part of the meaning, but the watcher of the shadow, and what it suggests."
Mahmoud Darwish in the preface to *Poésie: La terre nous est étroite.*

In your hands lies my translation of Volumes IV-VI of Chén Xiūyuán's *Jīn Guì Fāng Gē Kuò* 《金匱方歌括》(Formulas from the Golden Cabinet with Songs). Sabine Wilms, whose contribution in the field of Chinese medical translation is truly exceptional, beautifully translated the first three volumes, thus very large shoes were left to fill in the rendering and translation of the present volumes. Therefore, I owe Sabine a huge debt of gratitude for raising the bar so high, resulting in the constant evaluation of my own work.

The translation of a book of such importance to the field of Chinese medicine is no easy task, and could not have been done alone. I could not have completed the text nor been comfortable submitting it, if it were not for the meticulous editing and thorough reading by my teacher, colleague, and friend David Song (宋淳), to whom I owe an immense debt of gratitude for taking the time to assist in the editing of the book and having the patience to deal with my incessant questioning on Chinese medicine, philosophy, and traditional customs. Also instrumental in the editing of the text were Zhù Xiǎohuì (祝小惠), Qú Yàn (瞿雁), and Mark Gearing. Their knowledge in this field is truly remarkable and I cannot thank them enough.

The objective and yet the greatest challenge in translating texts like these is the ability to recreate someone else's work of art with fluidity and sensitivity, and bring creative energy and imagination to the work without losing the author's style, message or unique flavor. Therefore I have done my best to produce as close to a literal translation as possible, while maintaining clinical relevancy for modern-day practitioners. Extensive footnotes have been added in areas where term translations were altered or where I felt more information was needed.

For every formula in the book there is an accompanying song or poem, this is a traditional Chinese method used to aid memorization. Read aloud in Chinese, these songs have a rhythmic flow that is nearly impossible to recreate in English. The majority of the songs will clearly not rhyme, yet the most pertinent information for the formula will be found within.

Translator's Preface and Acknowledgments

The most-often quoted rule for high-quality translation was proposed by Yán Fù (嚴复) (1853–1921), one of the greatest translators of the late *Qīng* Dynasty and early Republican period. In his essay "*Tiān Yǎn Lùn* 《天演論》(Evolution and Ethics)," wrote that there are three fundamental challenges to overcome when translating: *xìn* 信 (fidelity), to the source text; *dá* 達 (clarity), of the target text; and *yǎ* 雅 (elegance). I have strived to address these challenges and it is my hope that this will be revealed in the work. As such, the translation of the Chinese language, specifically Classical Chinese medicine, can be subjective and open to interpretation. I have done my best to adhere to the original text, with careful consideration towards clinical relevancy.

As a student of the medical classics, primarily the writings of Zhāng Zhòngjǐng, I have also spent many years ardently studying the works and the many commentators on his works, primarily those of Chén Xiūyuán from his *Three Character Classic on Medical Studies* 《三字經》, to his *'Shallow' Commentaries* on the *Shāng Hán Lùn* and *Jīn Guì Yào Lüè* 《傷寒論淺注》,《金匮要略浅注》. Chén was a true student of the medical classics and was always quick to question and even criticize the work of others- who in his eyes, were steering far from the classics and inventing their own ideas without any true clinical relevancy. It is an absolute honor to have spent the last couple of years engulfed in this project translating a *Qīng* Dynasty commentary on one of the most important texts ever written. It has given me even greater insight into the true brilliance of not only this man, but also the brilliance of the clinicians who studied with him and offered numerous commentaries in this text, primarily his children and grandchildren. Chén had the incredible ability of turning rather obscure theories and ideas into real, tangible, and accessible skills one could utilize immediately. Thus I believe that Chén's work plays a valuable role in sharpening and increasing one's clinical skills in the modern-day clinic. This work should not be overlooked.

I want to give special thanks to the writers of the forewards: Z'ev Rosenberg, who is a pivotal force in Chinese medicine, a true scholar, a clinician and a person who was instrumental in my decision to become a practitioner of Chinese medicine and Húang Huáng, who has played an equally important role in bringing the teachings of the classics to the West through his many books, publications and overall enthusiasm and love for Classical Chinese medicine. I am truly honored to have this book begin with words from these great men.

Jonathan Schell at the Chinese Medicine Database has been a tremendous source of assistance and support during the process of translating this book. Jonathan's commitment was apparent in his eagerness to assist with difficult passages and his desire to make himself available in order to complete the text. Through the Database, Jonathan is playing an instrumental role in bringing these classics to life for English-speaking readers, and I am honored to have been a part of his mission to do so.

There are numerous other people who have offered tremendous support in this project but most notably I would like to thank Arnaud Versluys, Andrea Hansen, Polly Ambermoon, Michael Givens, Sharon Weizenbaum, Susan Chen, my family and especially my wife, Christine, for her devotion and commitment to support my work on the book even amidst the occasional chaos of our day-to-day lives. Last but certainly not least, I thank my daughters Sophie and Lila for their love and patience with their father during periods of total consumption by the text, and for their familiarity with the work of Zhāng Zhòngjǐng at such an early age.

Eran Even
Port Moody, British Columbia, Canada
July 2014

卷四
Volume Four

五臟風寒積聚方
Wǔ Zàng Fēng Hán Jī Jù Fāng

Formulas for Wind and Cold in the Five Viscera and Accumulations and Gatherings

旋覆花湯
Xuán Fù Huā Tāng
Inula Decoction

治肝著，其人常欲蹈其胸上，先未苦時，但欲飲熱者主之 。

A treatment for liver stickiness,[1] [where] the patient frequently desires to pound on their chest. Before the acute stage, only hot drinks are desired, [and this formula] rules it.

旋覆花（ 三兩 ）蔥（ 十四莖 ）新絳（ 少許 ）

xuán fù huā	旋覆花	9g
cōng [bái]	蔥	14 stems
xīn jiàng	新絳	a small amount

上三味，以水三升，煮取一升，頓服 。

Simmer the three ingredients above in 600ml of water until reduced to 200ml and remove the dregs. Take by drinking down in one gulp.

1. Wiseman translates the character *zhuó* 著 as fixity. Liver fixity: A disease pattern arising when liver qì and blood become stagnant and depressed. Liver fixity is characterized by glomus and oppression in the rib-side, in severe cases with pain and distension. (*A Practical Dictionary of Chinese Medicine*, second edition, Nigel Wiseman and Féng Yè (Paradigm Publications, 1999).

Song 歌曰:

肝著之人欲蹈胸，
肝氣著滯反行其氣於肺，所謂橫之病也。
胸者肺之位，欲按摩之以通其氣也。
熱湯一飲便輕鬆，
欲飲熱者，欲著之氣得熱則散。
覆花三兩蔥十四，
新絳通行少許從。
旋覆花咸溫下氣，新絳和血，蔥葉通陽。
新絳，查本草無此名。
按《說文》：絳，大赤也。
《左都賦》注：絳，草也，可以染色。
陶宏景曰：絳，茜草也。

A patient with liver stickiness desires to pound their chest;
liver qì stagnates adversely in the lung, and is therefore called a transverse disease.
The lung is located in the chest, and a desire to massage it, frees the qì.
Hot drinks can help one to relax,
as for the desire for warm drinks; the qì is about to be fixed, therefore heat can dissipate it,
nine grams of *xuán fù huā*, fourteen stems of *cōng bái*,
and *xīn jiàng* can slightly free and move.
***Xuán fù huā* warms and lowers qì, *xīn jiàng* harmonizes the blood, and *cōng bái* frees the yáng.**
There is no reference to *xīn jiàng* in the *Běn Cǎo*.
According to the *Shūo Wén*[2]: the character *jiàng* 絳 means a dark-red color.[3]
According to a comment in the *Zǔo Dū Fù*[4]: *jiàng*, is a leaf which is able to dye,
and according to Táo Hóngjǐng: *jiàng* refers to *qìan cǎo*.

2. *Shuō Wén Jiě Zì*《說文解字》, was an early second century A.D. (*Hàn* Dynasty) Chinese dictionary compiled by Xǔ Shèn 許慎.

3. Crimson.

4. Most likely a reference to the *Shǔ Dū Fù*《蜀都賦》(Shǔ Capitol Rhapsody), written by Zǔo Sī 左思, a renowned writer and poet of the western *Jìn* Dynasty.

麻仁丸

Má Rén Wán[5]

Hemp Seed Pill

歌見《傷寒》。

For the song, see the *Shāng Hán Lùn.*

治趺陽脈浮而濇，浮則胃氣強，濇則小便數，浮濇相搏，大便則堅，其脾為約，此丸主之。

When treating an instep yáng pulse, which is floating and rough, [bear in mind that the] floating reflects strong qì in the stomach, and the rough [quality] reflects frequent urination. The floating and rough struggle with each other, and the stool is hard, which means that the spleen is straitened.[6] This pill rules it.

麻子仁（二升）芍藥（半斤）枳實（半斤，炙）大黃（一斤，去皮）厚朴（一尺，炙，去皮）杏仁（一升，去皮尖，熬，別作脂）

má zǐ rén	麻子仁		400ml
sháo yào	芍藥		24g
zhǐ shí	枳實	honey-fried	24g
dà huáng	大黃	remove skin	48g
hòu pò	厚朴	honey-fried and skin removed	1 foot
xìng rén	杏仁	skin and tops removed, toast, remove the fat	200ml

上六味，蜜和丸，如梧桐子大，飲服十丸，日三服，漸加，以知為度。

---

5. In the *Shāng Hán Lùn*, this formula is called *Má Zǐ Rén Wán* 麻子仁丸.

6. "According to Chéng Wújǐ's 成無己 *Zhù Jiě Shāng Hán Lùn*《注解傷寒論》(The Annotated Cold Damage), "Straitened means constrained or to conserve resources." Chéng goes on to say "A strong stomach and weak spleen constrains the fluids, and prevents their distribution in the four directions. [Fluids] are only transported to the bladder, resulting in frequent urination and difficult defecation."

Process the six ingredients above into a powder and combine with refined honey to form pills the size of firmiana seeds.[7] Take ten pills with water, three doses per day. Gradually increase the number of pills until the stools are free.

Commentary 按:

脈浮者陽盛，脈濇者陰傷，脾為胃行其津液，陰傷則脾無所運矣。又約者弱也。脾弱不運，胃中谷食不化，則為積聚症也。餘義見《傷寒論》，不再贅。

[Here], the floating pulse signifies yáng exuberance, while the rough pulse indicates damage to yīn. The spleen serves to move fluids throughout the stomach, and when yīn is damaged, there is nothing for the spleen to move, resulting in weakness. When the spleen is weak and fails to move, there is non-transformation of food in the stomach, which leads to diseases of accumulation and gatherings. For further explanation of its meaning, see the *Shāng Hán Lùn.* It is superfluous to repeat it here.

7. *Wú tóng zǐ* 梧桐子 (firmiana seeds) are roughly 6-8mm in diameter, and were used as a reference point for the size of pills.

甘薑苓白朮湯

Gān Jiāng Líng Bái Zhú Tāng[8]

Licorice, Dried Ginger, Poria, and Ovate Atractylodes Decoction

一名腎著湯。

Also called "Kidney Stickiness Decoction."

治腎著之病，其人身體重，腰中冷，如坐水中，形如水狀，反不渴，小便自利，飲食如故，病屬下焦，身勞汗出，衣裏冷濕，久久得之，腰以下冷痛，腹重如帶五千錢者，此主之 。

A treatment for kidney stickiness[9] disease, in which the patient experiences generalized heaviness and lumbar coldness, as if they are sitting in water. Symptoms resemble those of water disease, yet there is no thirst, urination is uninhibited, and eating and drinking are normal. This means that the disease is in the lower burner. Physical taxation with sweating leads to cold and dampness in the clothes. Over an extended period of time [this] manifests with cold pain below the waist and abdominal heaviness as if carrying five thousand coins. This formula rules it.

甘草白朮（ 各二兩 ）乾薑茯苓（ 各四兩 ）

gān cǎo	甘草	6g
bái zhú	白朮	6g
gān jiāng	乾薑	12g
fú líng	茯苓	12g

上四味，以水五升，煮取三升，分溫三服，腰即溫 。

Simmer the four ingredients above in 1,000ml of water until reduced to 600ml. Divide and take warm in three doses, until the lower back feels warm.

8. Referred to as *Gān Cǎo Gān Jiāng Líng Zhú Tāng* 甘草乾薑苓朮湯 in the *Jīn Guì Yào Lüè*.

9. See footnote above. Kidney Fixity: cold pain and heaviness in the lumbar region that prevents normal turning and is exacerbated by yīn-type (dull, wet) weather, attributed to kidney vacuity, and cold-damp becoming "fixed" in the inner body. (*A Practical Dictionary of Chinese Medicine*, second edition, Nigel Wiseman and Féng Yè, Paradigm Publications, 1999).

Song 歌曰:

腰冷溶溶坐水泉，
帶脈束於腰間，
腎著則腰帶病，
故溶溶如坐水中狀。
腹中如帶五千錢，
朮甘二兩薑苓四，
寒濕同驅豈偶然？

Lumbar coldness as if sitting in gently flowing water springs.
The girdling vessel binds around the lower back.
With kidney stickiness there is disease in the waist,
which therefore brings the feeling as if one is sitting in water.
The abdomen feels as if it is carrying five thousand coins.
[With] six grams each of *bái zhú* and *gān cǎo*, and twelve of *gān jiāng* and *fú ling*,
is it by chance that both cold and dampness are expelled?

Quotation by Yóu Zàijīng[10] 尤在涇云:

寒濕之邪，不在腎之中臟，而在腎之外府，故其治不在溫腎以散寒，而在燠土以勝水。若用桂、附，則反傷腎之陰矣。

Cold-damp evils are not located in the kidney viscera, but in the external dwelling of the kidneys. Therefore, treatment need not involve warming the kidneys in order to dissipate cold, but to warm[11] the earth in order to prevail over water. If *guì zhī*, or *fù zǐ* were used, then kidney yīn would be damaged!

10. Yóu Zàijīng 尤在涇 (??-1749), was a well-known *Qíng* Dynasty scholar-physician from Chángzhōu (modern day Wú county in Jiāngsū province), who wrote several commentaries on *Hàn* Dynasty medical literature, including the *Jīn Guì Yì* 金匮翼 (Appendices to the Golden Cabinet).

11. The character *yù* 燠 here means warm or warmth.

痰飲咳嗽方
Tán Yǐn Ké Sòu Fāng

Formulas for Phlegm-Rheum Cough

苓桂朮甘湯
Líng Guì Zhú Gān Tāng
Poria, Cinnamon Twig, Ovate Atractylodes, and Licorice Decoction

歌見《傷寒》。

For the song, see the *Shāng Hán Lùn.*

治心下有痰飲，胸脅支滿，目眩者 。

A treatment for phlegm-rheum below the heart with propping fullness in the chest and rib-side, [as well as] dizzy vision.

茯苓（ 四兩 ）桂枝（ 三兩 ）白朮（ 三兩 ）甘草（ 二兩 ）

fú líng	茯苓	12g
guì zhī	桂枝	9g
bái zhú	白朮	9g
gān cǎo	甘草	6g

上四味，以水六升，煮取三升，分溫三服，小便則利 。

Simmer the four ingredients above in 1,200ml of water until reduced to 600ml. Divide and take warm in three doses, until the urine is uninhibited.

Commentary by [Chén] Xīndiǎn[12] 次孫男心典稟按:

心下者，脾之部位也。飲凌於脾，致脾弱不輸，不能制水，則生痰矣，故曰心下有痰飲也。胸乃人身之太空，為陽氣往來之道路，飲邪彌漫於胸，盈滿於脅，蔽其君陽，溢於支絡，故曰胸脅支滿也。動則水氣蕩漾，其變態無常，或頭旋轉，目冒眩，心動悸諸症，皆隨其所作也。

The area below the heart is the location of the spleen. When encroached by rheum, the spleen becomes weak and is unable to transport and dam water, which invariably results in the generation of phlegm! Therefore, we call this phlegm-rheum below the heart. The chest is the body's great space, which serves as a path for yáng qì to travel. When evil rheum pervades the chest and fills the rib-sides, sovereign yáng becomes concealed, and [rheum] seeps into the branch collaterals. This, we call propping fullness in the chest and rib-sides. When stirred, water qì is flushed out, overflows and becomes abnormal. [This manifests] with possible vertigo, visual veiling dizziness, and heart palpitations, which always vary according to [the water's] location [in the body].

主以苓桂朮甘湯者，以茯苓為君，蓋以苓者令也，使治節之令行，而水可從令而下耳；桂枝振心陽以退其群陰，如離照當空則陰霾全消，而天日復明也；白朮補中土以修其堤岸，使水無泛濫之虞；更以甘草助脾氣轉輸以交上下，靡治節行，心陽振，土氣旺，轉輸速，而水有下行之勢，無上凌之患矣。

The ruling formula, *Líng Guì Zhú Gān Tāng* uses *fú líng* as the sovereign. Now, *fú líng* is the commander, which orders the management and regulation of movement, for which water can follow and descend. *Guì zhī* vitalizes heart yáng in order to reduce the multitude of yīn, and as it departs accordingly and empties, the haze will completely disperse, and the brightness of both heaven and the sun will return. *Bái zhú* supplements center earth in order to build its embankment and prevent the flooding of water. Furthermore, *gān cǎo* assists spleen qì in its activity of movement in order to create interaction between the upper and lower body. Ordinarily when there is management and regulation of movement, heart yáng is roused, earth qì flourishes, shifts, and transports quickly, and water has the power to descend downwards, so there is no worry of [water] ascending and encroaching on [the upper body].

12. Chén Xīndiǎn was Chén Xiūyuán's grandson, and the eldest son of Chén Yuánxī. The character *cì* 次, which means second in this context refers to Chén Yuánxī, who is Chén's second child, therefore the above can also be translated as "commentary by [Chén's] grandson Chén Xīndiǎn [from his] second child."

腎氣丸

Shèn Qì Wán

Kidney Qì Pill

歌見婦人雜病。

For the song, see [the section on] "Miscellaneous Gynecological Diseases."

治短氣有微飲，當從小便去之，苓桂朮甘湯主之；此丸亦主之 。

Treatment for shortness of breath with mild rheum, [which] should be eliminated through urination. *Líng Guì Zhú Gān Tāng* rules it. *Shèn Qì Wán* also rules.

乾地黃（ 八兩 ）山藥 山茱萸（ 各四兩 ）澤瀉 牡丹皮 茯苓（ 各三兩 ）桂枝 附子（ 炮 。各一兩 ）

gān dì huáng	乾地黃		24g
shān yào	山藥		12g
shān zhū yú	山茱萸		12g
zé xiè	澤瀉		9g
mǔ dān pí	牡丹皮		9g
fú líng	茯苓		9g
guì zhī	桂枝		3g
fù zǐ	附子	blast-fried	3g

上八味末之，煉蜜和丸梧子大，酒下十五丸，加至二十五丸，日再服 。

Process the eight ingredients above into a powder and combine with refined honey to form pills the size of firmiana seeds. Swallow fifteen pills [per dose] with liquor, increasing the dosage to a maximum of twenty-five pills, two doses per day.

Commentary by [Chén] Xīnlán[13] 次孫男心蘭稟按:

微者，不顯之謂也。飲，水也。微飲者，猶陰霾四布，細雨輕飛之狀。阻於胸中。蔽其往來之氣，故曰短氣。有微飲者，謂微飲阻其氣路也。經云：呼出心與肺，吸入肝與腎。若心肺之陽虛，則不能行水化氣，用苓桂朮甘湯振心陽崇土以防御之，使天日明而陰霾散，則氣化行矣。若腎虛而水泛，則吸引無權，當用腎氣丸補腎行水，使腎氣足，則能通腑而化氣，氣化[14]則水道通矣。余解見婦人雜病，不再贅。

Mild refers to something that is not prominent. Rheum is water. Mild rheum can be likened to a state of gentle drizzling or the dispersion of mist. When it is obstructed in the chest, the movement of qì is hindered, and this is referred to as shortness of breath. Therefore, with mild rheum one can say that the path for qì [movement] is obstructed. The classics say that exhalation is related to the heart and lungs, while inhalation is related to the liver and kidneys. If the heart or lungs suffer from yáng vacuity, they would be unable to move water or transform qì. *Líng Guì Zhú Gān Tāng* is used to vitalize heart yáng and strengthen [the] earth, in order to prevent [further rheum from forming], thus enabling the brightness of the sun in the sky to dissipate the mist. Only then will qì transformation[15] occur. If there is a kidney vacuity with flooding of water, resulting in failure to inhale, one should use *Shèn Qì Wán* in order to supplement the kidneys, move water, and cause the kidney qì to be sufficient, which will free the bowels and transform qì. With qì transformation, the water pathways will be clear! For my explanation, see [the section on] "Miscellaneous Gynecological Diseases." It is superfluous to repeat it here.

13. Chén Xīnlán was Chén Xiūyuán's grandson, and the second-eldest son of Chén Yuánxī. See footnote above.

14. In an edition published by the *Wěi Wén Táng Cáng Bǎn* 緯文堂藏板, *huà qì* "化氣" is written as *qì huà* "氣化."

15. Qì transformation: The movement, mutation, and conversion of qì. Qì transformation refers to the processes by which the six qì (essence, qì, liquid, humor, blood, and vessels [or pulse] produce each other and convert from one another. (*Practical Dictionary of Chinese Medicine*, Wiseman et al., p. 486).

甘遂半夏湯

Gān Suì Bàn Xià Tāng

Kansui and Pinellia Decoction

治脈伏，其人欲自利，利反快，雖利，心下續堅滿，此為留飲欲去故也，此主之。

A treatment for a hidden pulse, where the patient is about to have spontaneous diarrhea, and experiences gratification following the diarrhea, [yet] continues [to have] hardness and fullness below the heart. This is due to lodged rheum, which is about to be eliminated. This [formula] rules it.

甘遂（大者三枚）半夏（十二枚，以水一升，煮取半升，去滓）芍藥（五枚）甘草（如指大[16]一枚，炙）

gān suì	甘遂		3 large pcs
bàn xià	半夏	boiled in 200ml of water until reduced to 100ml. Remove the dregs.	12 pcs
sháo yào	芍藥		5 pcs
gān cǎo	甘草	honey-fried, one large finger sized pc.	1 pc

上四味，以水二升，煮取半升，去滓，以蜜半升和藥汁，煎取八合，頓服之。

Simmer the four ingredients above in 400ml of water until reduced to 100ml. Remove the dregs, and decoct again with 100ml of honey until reduced to 160ml. Take in a single dose.

16. In a large-print edition of the book, published by the *Wěi Wén Táng Cáng Bǎn* 緯文堂藏板, “one piece, honey fried” is written.

Song 歌曰:

滿從利減續還來，
去者自去，續者自續。
甘遂三枚芍五枚，
十二枚夏指大草，
水煎加蜜法雙該。

Fullness is reduced following diarrhea, yet continues and returns.
When [fullness] is eliminated diarrhea will be as well,
and when [fullness] continues, so too will the diarrhea.
[In this case use] three pieces of *gān suì*, and five of *sháo yào*.
Twelve pieces *bàn xià*, and *gān cǎo* the size of a finger.
Add honey to the decoction and [use the method] of double cooking mentioned above.

Quotation by Yóu Zàijīng 尤在涇云:

雖利，心下續堅滿者，未盡之飲複注心下也。然雖未盡而有欲去之勢，故以甘遂、半夏因其勢而導之；甘遂與甘草遂相反而同用之者，蓋欲其一戰而留飲盡去，因相激而相成也；芍藥、白蜜，不特安中，抑緩藥毒耳。

Although there is diarrhea, there continues to be hardness and fullness below the heart. Rheum which has not yet been terminated pours below the heart. However, although the rheum has not yet been completely expelled, *gān suì* and *bàn xià* are used to provide the momentum to guide it out. *Gān suì* and *gān cǎo* when used together are [traditionally known] to clash [with one another], but using them this way [one] is able to eliminate lodged rheum in one battle, [thus we sometimes] rely on mutually restraining [medicinals], which can assist each other in order to achieve this outcome. *Sháo yào* and *bái mì* not only quiet the center, but also control and moderate the toxicity of the medicinals.

十棗湯

Shí Zǎo Tāng

Ten Jujubes Decoction

歌方見《傷寒》。

For the song, see the *Shāng Hán Lùn.*

脈沉而弦者，懸飲內痛，病懸飲者，此湯主之。

Deep and wiry pulses indicate suspended rheum with interior pain.[17] For suspended rheum, this decoction rules it.

芫花（熬）甘遂大戟（各等分）

yuán huā	芫花	boiled, equal amounts
gān suì	甘遂	
dà jǐ	大戟	

上三味，搗篩，以水一升五合，先煮肥大棗十枚，取八合，去滓，內藥末。強人服一錢匕，羸人服半錢。平旦溫服之。不下者，明日更服加半錢，得快之後，糜粥自養。

Pound and sift equal amounts of the three ingredients above. In 300ml of water, first boil ten plump pieces of *dà zǎo* until reduced to 160ml. Remove the dregs and add the medicinal powder. Give stronger patients one *qián*-spoonful, and a half spoonful for weak patients. Take warm early in the morning. If there is no precipitation, take another half *qián* the next day. After the bowels are free, rice gruel should be taken for nourishment.

17. Interior pain: pain extending into the chest and rib-sides while coughing.

Commentary by [Chén] Yuánxī[18] 男元犀按:

脈沉主裏，弦主飲，飲水凝結，懸於胸膈之間，致咳引內痛也。懸飲既成，緩必滋蔓，急用十棗湯直達病所，不嫌其峻。意謂始成而即攻之，使水飲下趨而無結痛之患，所謂毒藥去病者是也；若畏其猛而不敢用，必遷延而成痼疾矣。

A deep pulse [is] ruled [by] the interior; a wiry pulse [is] ruled [by] rheum. Water-rheum is congealed, bound, and suspended in the space between the chest and the diaphragm, causing a cough and leading to interior pain. Since suspended rheum has formed, we must prevent its growth and spread, therefore, *Shí Zǎo Tāng* is swiftly used to directly outthrust it from the disease location, and [one should not] be suspicious of its harshness. The significance here is that once [water-rheum] has begun to develop, it should be immediately attacked, causing water-rheum to converge downwards, preventing the suffering from binding pain. This is achieved by using toxic medicinals to eliminate the disease. If one fears this fierce method and does not dare to use it, this will most certainly prolong [the disease], which will inevitably become an intractable condition.

18. In the first three volumes of the text, Chén Yuánxī is simply referred to as Yuánxī; however in the present volumes, he is now referred to as [Nán] Yuánxī. In this context Nán 男 simply means 'a male son.' It is unclear why the text has changed in the present volumes, but from here on, he will simply be referred to as [Chén] Yuánxī.

大青龍湯

Dà Qīng Lóng Tāng

Major Blue-Green Dragon Decoction

歌見《傷寒》。

For the song, see the *Shāng Hán Lùn.*

麻黄（六兩，去節）桂枝（二兩，去皮）甘草（二兩，炙）杏仁（四十枚，去皮尖）生薑（三兩，切）大棗（十二枚）石膏（如雞子大，碎）

má huáng	麻黄	knots removed	18g
guì zhī	桂枝	bark removed	6g
gān cǎo	甘草	honey-fried	6g
xìng rén	杏仁	skin and tops removed	14 pits
shēng jiāng	生薑	cut	9g
dà zǎo	大棗	broken	12 pcs
shí gāo	石膏	smashed	1 pc the size of a chicken egg

上七味，以水九升，先煮麻黄，減二升，去上沫，內諸藥，煮取三升，去滓，溫服一升，取微似汗。汗多者，溫粉粉之。

For the seven ingredients above, use 1,800ml of water. First boil the *má huáng* and reduce the water by 400ml. Remove the foam collecting on the surface and add the other ingredients. Simmer until reduced to 600ml, remove the dregs, and take 200ml warm, until a mild sweat is obtained. If there is copious sweating, apply warm rice powder [to the exterior of the body].

小青龍湯

Xiǎo Qīng Lóng Tāng

Minor Blue-Green Dragon Decoction

歌見《傷寒》。

For the song, see the *Shāng Hán Lùn*.

治病溢飲者，當發其汗，大青龍湯主之；小青龍湯亦主之。

When treating spillage-rheum disease, sweat should be promoted. *Dà Qīng Lóng Tāng* rules it. *Xiǎo Qīng Lóng Tāng* also rules it.

麻黃（三兩，去節）芍藥（三兩）五味子（半升）乾薑（三兩）甘草（三兩，炙）細辛（三兩）桂枝（三兩，去皮）半夏（半升，洗）

má huáng	麻黃	knots removed	9g
sháo yào	芍藥		9g
wǔ wèi zǐ	五味子		100ml
gān jiāng	乾薑		9g
gān cǎo	甘草	honey-fried	9g
xì xīn	細辛		9g
guì zhī	桂枝	bark removed	9g
bàn xià	半夏	washed	100ml

上八味，以水一斗，先煮麻黃，減二升，去上沫，內諸藥，煮取三升，去滓，溫服一升。

For the eight ingredients above use 2,000ml of water. First boil the *má huáng* and reduce the water by 400ml. Remove the foam collecting on the surface, and add the other ingredients. Boil until reduced to 600ml, remove the dregs, and take 200ml warm.

Commentary by [Chén] Yuánxī 男元犀按：

師云：飲水流行歸於四肢，當汗而不汗出，身體疼重，謂之溢飲，故病溢飲者，以得汗為出路。然飲既流溢，亦隨人之臟氣寒熱而化。飲從熱化，故立大青龍湯辛涼發汗以行水；飲從寒化，故立小青龍湯辛溫發汗以行水。二方並列，用者當酌其宜焉。

The master says: [when] water-rheum spreads into the four extremities, there should be sweating, yet there is none, [and this is] accompanied by pain and heaviness in the body; [this] is called spillage-rheum. As this is a spillage-rheum disease, [one must] obtain a sweat to remove it. Since rheum has already flowed and seeped, it can also be transformed alongside heat and cold of the body's visceral qì. If rheum has transformed to heat, one can use the acrid, cool, sweat-effusing *Dà Qīng Lóng Tāng* in order to move water, and if rheum has been transformed to cold, then acrid, warm, sweat-effusing *Xiǎo Qīng Lóng Tāng* can be given to disinhibit water. One must always consider when it is most appropriate to use either of these two contrasting formulas.

木防己湯
Mù Fáng Jĭ Tāng
Cocculi Decoction

治膈間支飲，其人喘滿，心下痞堅，面色黧黑，其脈沉緊，得之數十日，醫吐下之不愈，此湯主之。虛者即愈，實者三日復發。復與不愈者，宜此湯去石膏加茯苓芒硝湯主之。

A treatment for propping-rheum, manifesting with panting, fullness, glomus and hardness below the heart, a soot-black facial complexion, and a deep-tight pulse. This can last for several days and does not resolve following ejection or purgation. This formula rules it. A vacuity pattern[19] will resolve immediately, while a repletion pattern[20] will start again after three days. Applying the same prescription will not be effective. [Here] it is suitable to give *Mù Fáng Jĭ Tāng Qù Shí Gāo Jiā Fú Líng Máng Xiāo Tāng.*

木防己（三兩）石膏（如雞子大二枚）桂枝（二兩）人參（四兩）

mù fáng jĭ	木防己	9g
shí gāo	石膏	2 pcs (the size of a large chicken egg)
guì zhī	桂枝	6g
rén shēn	人參	12g

上四味，以水六升，煮取二升，分溫再服。

Simmer the four ingredients above in 1,200ml of water until reduced to 400ml. Divide and take warm in two doses.

Song 歌曰:

喘滿痞堅面色黧，
己三桂二四參施，
膏枚二個如雞子，
辛苦寒溫各適宜。

19. A vacuity pattern, in this case is characterized by a 'soft' glomus.
20. The repletion pattern, is characterized by glomus and hardness below the heart.

[With] panting, fullness, hard glomus, and a soot-black facial complexion,
[use] nine grams of ***mù fáng jǐ***, six grams ***guì zhī***, ***rén shēn*** at twelve,
and two pieces of ***shí gāo*** the size of a chicken egg.
[The use of] acrid, bitter, cold, and warm [medicinals] is appropriate.

Commentary by [Chén] Yuánxī 男元犀按：

防己入手太陰肺，肺主氣，氣化而水自行矣；桂枝入足太陽膀胱，膀胱主水，水行結散，則心下痞堅可除矣。然病得數十日之久，又經吐下，可知胃陰傷而虛氣逆。故用人參以生既傷之陰，石膏以鎮虛逆之氣，陰復逆平，則喘滿面黧自愈矣。此方治其本來，救其失誤，面面俱到。

Fáng jǐ enters the hand tàiyīn lung [channel]. The lungs rule qì, and when qì transforms, water moves on its own. *Guì zhī* enters the foot tàiyáng bladder [channel]. The bladder rules water, and when water moves, the bind will dissipate and the hard glomus below the heart can be eliminated. Since the disease has lasted for more than several tens of days and ejection and purgation have been used, [we] know that stomach yīn has been damaged, and vacuous qì is running counterflow. Therefore [in this case], ***rén shēn*** is used in order to generate the already damaged yīn. ***Shí gāo*** is used to suppress the vacuous counterflow of qì. Once yīn is returned to a balanced state, the panting, fullness, and soot-black facial complexion will spontaneously resolve. This formula treats the original [problem] and rescues from the erroneous [treatment], dealing with the entire situation [at hand].

木防己去石膏加茯苓芒硝湯

Mù Fáng Jǐ Qù Shí Gāo Jiā Fú Líng Máng Xiāo Tāng

Cocculi Decoction minus Gypsum plus Poria and Mirabilite Decoction

木防己（ 三兩 ）桂枝（ 二兩 ）茯苓人參（ 各四兩 ）芒硝（ 三合 ）

mù fáng jǐ	木防己	9g
guì zhī	桂枝	6g
fú líng	茯苓	12g
rén shēn	人參	12g
máng xiāo	芒硝	60ml

上五味，以水六升，煮取二升，去滓，內芒硝，再微煎，分溫再服，微利則愈。

Simmer the five ingredients above in 1,200ml of water until reduced to 400ml, and remove the dregs. Add the *máng xiāo* and return to a gentle boil. Divide and take warm in two doses. Once there is slight diarrhea, recovery will ensue.

Song 歌曰:

四兩苓加不用膏，
芒硝三合展奇韜；
氣行復聚知為實，
以軟磨堅自不勞。

Twelve grams *fú líng*, for there is no need for *shí gāo*,
[add] 60ml of *máng xiāo*, and a wonderful strategy is established;
[when] qì moves [yet] accumulations re-gather, we know [it is due] to repletion,
[and using] softness to wear out the hardness, will surely not over-exert.

Quotation by Wèi Niàntíng[21] **魏念庭云：**

前方去石膏加芒硝者，以其邪既散而復聚，則有堅定之物留作包囊，故以堅投堅而不破者，即以軟投堅而即破也。加茯苓者，亦引飲下行之用耳。

This is the previous formula [*Mù Fáng Jǐ Tāng*] with *shí gāo* removed and *máng xiāo* added. Dissipated evil has gathered once again, [and] there is hardness remaining as a fixed membrane. Therefore, [in this case] using hardness to cast away hardness would not break [it], but using softness to dispose of hardness breaks it. The addition of *fú líng* functions to move and guide rheum downwards.

21. A physician from the *Qīng* Dynasty who composed the *Jīn Guì Yào Lüè Fāng Lùn Běn Yì*《金匱要略方論本義》(Root Meaning of the Formulas and Essays in the Golden Cabinet).

澤瀉湯

Zé Xiè Tāng

Alisma Decoction

治心下有支飲，其人苦冒眩者，主之。

A treatment for propping-rheum below the heart, where the person suffers from veiling dizziness; [this formula] rules it.

澤瀉（五兩）白朮（二兩）

zé xiè	澤瀉	15g
bái zhú	白朮	6g

上二味，以水二升，煮取一升，分溫再服。

Simmer the two ingredients above in 400ml of water until reduced to 200ml. Divide and take warm in two doses.

Song 歌曰:

清陽之位飲邪乘，
眩冒頻頻苦不勝；
澤五為君朮二兩，
補脾制水有奇能。

The location of clear yáng has been overwhelmed by the presence of rheum evil,
causing [one to] suffer from frequent veiling dizziness which is difficult to endure;
fifteen grams of the sovereign *zé xiè* and six of *bái zhú*,
have the special ability of supplementing the spleen and controlling water.

Commentary by Lín Lǐfēng[22] **受業林禮豐按:**

心者，陽中之陽。頭者，諸陽之會。人之有陽氣，猶天之有日也。天以日而光明，猶人之陽氣會於頭而目能明視也。夫心下有支飲，則飲邪上蒙於心，心陽被遏不能上會於巔，故有頭冒目眩之病。仲師特下一"苦"字，是水陰之氣盪漾於內，而冒眩之苦有莫可言傳者，故主澤瀉陽。蓋澤瀉氣味甘寒，生於水中，得水陰之氣而能利水，一莖直上，能從下而上，同氣相求，領水陰之氣以下走，然猶恐水氣下而復上，故用白朮之甘溫，崇土制水者以諸之，猶治水者之必筑堤防也。古聖用方之妙，有如此者。

The heart is yáng within yáng; the head is the gathering place of all yáng. Humans have yáng qì, as heaven has the sun. Heaven by means of the sun is bright; as such, humans' yáng qì gathers in the head and eyes, providing bright vision. When there is propping-rheum below the heart, water-rheum will ascend and cloud the heart, obstructing heart yáng, which is [then] unable to gather at the top of the head, causing dizziness and dizzy vision. Master Zhòng used the character *kǔ* [苦] to convey the suffering of dizziness, [resulting from] the qì of water yīn agitating and flowing into the interior. This is ruled by *Zé Xiè Tāng*. The qì and flavor of *zé xiè* is sweet and cold, and since it grows in water, it obtains the qì of water yīn, [so] it is able to disinhibit water. [Similar to the way] the stalk ascends vertically, it can [help] bring the qì together from the bottom to the top and guide the qì of water yīn in its downward movement. However if one fears [that the] water qì will ascend again after it has [already] descended, then use sweet and warm *bái zhú* to venerate earth and restrain the various forms of water. Similarly by treating water, [one] will build an embankment. The ancient sages were very clever in using formulas like these.

今人反以澤瀉利水伐腎，多服傷目之說疑之。其說創於宋元諸醫，而李時珍、張景岳、李士材、汪讱庵輩和之，貽害至今弗熄。然天下人信李時珍之《本草》者，殆未讀《神農本草經》耶？余先業師《神農本經小注》最詳，願業斯道者，三復之而後可。

People nowadays are administering copious amounts of *zé xiè* to disinhibit water and quell the kidneys, which damages the objective [of this] doctrine and [creates] doubt [of its effectiveness]. This doctrine began with the physicians of the *Sóng*[23] and *Yuàn*[24] dynasties, as well as contempo-

22. Lín Lǐfēng was believed to be a student of Chén Xiǔyuán. The characters 受業 can be translated as: to receive instructions, to study, to learn from a master, or as a first pronoun, such as I, or your student, and is often used as a title by a teachers' disciple. I have opted to translate this as the latter, as opposed to Commentary by I [your student] Lín Lǐfēng.

23. *Sòng* Dynasty (960–1179 A.D.).

24. *Yuán* (Mongol) Dynasty (1260–1368 A.D.).

raries such as Lǐ Shízhēn,[25] Zhāng Jǐngyuè,[26] Lǐ Shìcái,[27] and Wāng Rènān,[28] who have left a legacy which has yet to die even to the present day. Even though people of the world trust the words of Lǐ Shízhēn's *Běn Cǎo,* why have almost [none of them] read the *Shén Nóng Běn Cǎo Jīng*? My passed[29] master's copy of the classic was annotated with extreme detail, and it is my hope that one follows this way in their course of study, repeatedly returning to [the classic].

25. Lǐ Shízhēn (1518–1593), *Míng* botanist and pharmacologist, as well as the author of the *Běn Cǎo Gāng Mù* 《本草綱目》(Compendium of medical herbs).

26. Late *Míng* Dynasty physician who wrote several books including the *Běn Cǎo Zhèng* 《本草正》(Rectification of the Materia Medica).

27. *Míng* Dynasty physician who wrote several books including the *Nèi Jīng Zhī Yāo* 《内經知要》(Essential Knowledge from the Inner Classic).

28. Wāng Áng (1615–1694), Late *Míng* and early *Qīng* Dynasty physician who wrote the *Běn Cǎo Bèi Yào* 《本草備要》(Essentials of the Materia Medica).

29. This refers to one of Chén's former masters who had died, and Chén was using this master's copy of the *Shén Nóng Běn Cǎo Jīng.*

厚朴大黃湯

Hòu Pò Dà Huáng Tāng

Magnolia Bark and Rhubarb Decoction

治支飲胸滿者，此湯主之。

When treating propping-rheum with chest fullness, this decoction rules.

厚朴（ 一尺 ）大黃（ 六兩 ）枳實（ 四枚 ）

hòu pò	厚朴	1 foot
dà huáng	大黃	18g
zhǐ shí	枳實	4 pcs

上三味，以水五升，煮取二升，分溫再服。

Simmer the three ingredients above in 1,000ml of water until reduced to 400ml. Divide and take warm in two doses.

Song 歌曰:

胸為陽位似天空，
支飲填胸滿不通；
尺朴為君調氣分，
四枚枳實六黃攻。

The chest is the position of yáng, which resembles the sky.
Propping-rheum fills the chest causing stoppage with fullness.
A foot of the sovereign *hòu pò* harmonizes the qì aspect,
and four pieces of *zhǐ* [*shí*] and eighteen grams of [*dà*] *huáng* attack.

Commentary by [Chén] Yuánxī 元犀按:

支飲者，有支派之別也。胸乃陽氣之道路，飲為陰邪，言胸滿者，乃陰佔陽位，填塞胸中而作滿也。君以厚朴者，味苦性溫，為氣分之藥，苦降溫開，使陽氣通，則胸中之飲化矣；枳實形圓臭香，香以醒脾，圓主旋轉，故用以為佐；繼以大黃直決地道，地道通，則飲邪有不順流而下出哉？

There are various branches [types] of propping-rheum. The chest is the pathway of yáng qì; rheum is a yīn evil. When we say "chest fullness" this is [due to] yīn occupying the position of yáng, and filling the chest with cold causing fullness. The sovereign is *hòu pò*, which is bitter in flavor, and warm in nature, and is a medicinal [which works] on the qì aspect. Its bitter [flavor] descends, while its warmth opens, allowing for the freeing of yáng qì, which then transforms rheum in the chest. *Zhǐ shí* is round in shape, and aromatic in fragrance. Its fragrance awakens the spleen, and its roundness rules rotation; therefore it is used as the assistant. *Dà huáng* is then used to directly clear the pathway. Once this path is free, how can rheum evil not have a favorable flow [in order to] be eliminated downwards?

Additional Commentary 又按:

小承氣湯是氣藥為臣，此湯是氣藥為君，其意以氣行而水亦行。意深矣。三物湯、小承氣湯與此湯藥品俱同，其分兩、主治不同，學者宜細心研究。

In *Xiǎo Chéng Qì Tāng* the qì medicinals are the ministers. In this decoction the qì medicinals are the sovereigns. The intention is that when qì moves, water will also move. This is a profound significance indeed! The medicinals in *Sǎn Wù Tāng*, *Xiǎo Chéng Qì Tāng*, and this decoction are all the same, only differentiated by three grams, yet their primary treatments are different. Students must be attentive [to these facts], and study meticulously.

葶藶大棗瀉肺湯

Tíng Lì Dà Zǎo Xiè Fèi Tāng

Lepidium/Descurainiae and Jujube Lung-Draining Decoction[30]

歌見肺癰。

For the song, see [the section on] "Lung Welling-Abscesses."

支飲不得息，此主之。

For propping-rheum with an inability to breath, this [formula] rules it.

Commentary by [Chén Yuán] Xī 犀按:

肺主氣，為出入之路。師云：支飲不得息者，乃飲邪壅肺，填塞氣路矣。方用葶藶洩肺氣以開之，大棗補脾土以納之，則氣息得矣。

The lungs rule qì, and are the road from which it exits and enters. The master has said, with propping-rheum, there is an inability to breathe, [this is] due to evil rheum congesting the lung, which obstructs the path of qì. The formula uses *tíng lì* to drain lung qì in order to open [it], and *dà zǎo* to supplement spleen earth to promote absorption, after which one is able to breathe.

30. Refer to page 169 of volume 1 for further information.

小半夏湯
Xiǎo Bàn Xià Tāng
Minor Pinellia Decoction

治嘔家本渴，渴者為欲解，今反不渴，心下有支飲故也，此湯主之。

A treatment for vomiting patients who are supposed to be thirsty; thirst indicates that the condition is on the verge of resolving. An absence of thirst indicates propping-rheum below the heart, and this decoction rules it.

半夏（一升）生薑（半斤）

bàn xià	半夏	200ml
shēng jiāng	生薑	24g

上二味，以水七升，煮取一升半，分溫再服。

Simmer the two ingredients above in 1,400ml of water until reduced to 300ml. Divide and take warm in two doses.

Song 歌曰:

嘔家見渴飲當除，
飲以嘔去，故渴。
不渴應知支飲居，
飲能制燥，今以不渴，
知心下有支飲。
半夏一升薑八兩，
源頭探得病根鋤。

In vomiting patients who are thirsty, rheum must [have been] eliminated.
When rheum and vomiting are gone, there is thirst.
With an absence of thirst, we know that propping-rheum still resides.
Rheum is able to restrain dryness and now there is an absence of thirst,
so we know that there is propping-rheum below the heart.

200ml of *bàn xià*, and twenty-four grams of [*shēng*] *jiāng*
[are able to] get deep and eliminate the source of the disease.

Commentary by [Chén] Yuánxī 男元犀按：

《神農本草經》載半夏之功治甚大，仲師各方，無不遵法用之。凡嘔者，必加此味。元明後，誤認為治痰專藥，遂有用朴硝水浸者；有用皂角角水及薑水浸者；有用白芥子和醋浸者，市中用烏梅、甘草、青鹽等制造者，更不堪入藥；近日通用水煮，乘熱以白礬拌曬切片者，皆失其本性，不能安胃止嘔。

It is recorded in the *Shén Nóng Běn Cǎo Jīng* that the treatment functions of *bàn xià* are quite large and, without exception, each one of Master Zhòng's[31] formulas observe these methods and uses. In all [cases] of vomiting, this medicinal must be added. Following the *Yuán* and *Míng* dynasties it was falsely believed to be a medicinal, that specifically treats phlegm, and has subsequently been used steeped in impure mirabilite (Natrii Sulfas Non-Purus) water, steeped in *zào jiǎo* water, *shēng jiāng* water, and with *bái jiè zǐ* and vinegar. Several markets now use *wū méi*, *gān cǎo*, salt, and various other substances in the manufacturing process rendering it inefficient for medical use. Currently it is common practice to boil [*bàn xià*], mix it with alum, sundry and slice. All these [methods] create the loss of the medicinals original nature, and eliminate the function of calming the stomach and stopping vomiting.

宜從古法，以湯泡七次，去涎用之，或畏其麻口，以薑汁、甘草水浸透心，洗淨曬乾，再以清水浸三日，每日換水，蒸熟曬乾用之。支飲之症，嘔而不渴者，旁支之飲未盡也。用小半夏湯者，重在生薑散旁支之飲，半夏降逆安胃，合之為滌飲下行之用。神哉！

Instead, one should observe and follow the ancient method of boiling seven times and removing the foam, and if [one] fears mouth numbness, then soak with ginger juice, or *gān cǎo* water. Wash clean, dry in the sun, and then steep in clear water for three days. The water should be changed daily, and afterwards, steam dry. In propping-rheum diseases, with vomiting and an absence of thirst, the propping-rheum has not yet been completely eliminated. In *Xiǎo Bàn Xià Tāng*, the key point is the use of *shēng jiāng* to dissipate propping-rheum. *Bàn xià* downbears counterflow and calms the stomach, and together these [two medicinals] serve to flush away rheum and cause downward movement. Magical!!

31. Zhāng Zhòngjǐng.

己椒藶黃丸

Jǐ Jiāo Lì Huáng Wán

Fangji, Zanthoxylum Seed, Tingli, and Rhubarb Pill

治腹滿，口舌乾燥，此腸間有水氣，此方主之。

A treatment for abdominal fullness, where [there is] thirst with a dry mouth and tongue. This indicates water qì in the intestines, and this formula rules it.

防己椒目葶藶大黃（各一兩）

fáng jǐ	防己	3g
jiāo mù	椒目	3g
tíng lì	葶藶	3g
dà huáng	大黃	3g

上四味末之，蜜丸如梧子大，先食飲服一丸，日三服，稍增，口中有津液。渴者，加芒硝半兩。

Process the four ingredients above into a powder and combine with honey to form pills the size of firmiana seeds. Take one pill before meals, three times daily. Gradually increase the dosage until salivation occurs. If the patient is thirsty, add 1.5g of *máng xiāo*.

Song 歌曰:

腸中有水口帶乾，
水既聚於下，則無復潤於上，
後即水飲之入，皆趨於下，
不能滋其燥，且以益其滿矣。
腹裏為腸按部觀，
腹裏為大小二腸部位，
大腸主津液，今作滿，
為水氣所傷，
則津液不能上達於口舌，

故乾燥。
椒己藶黃皆一兩，
蜜丸飲服日三餐。

Water in the intestines, and the region of the mouth is dry.
Water has gathered in the lower body, and fails to return and moisten the upper.
After water-rheum has entered, it tends to [descend] towards the lower,
being unable to enrich the dryness, and even benefiting fullness!
The location of the intestines is within the abdomen.
Both the large and small intestines reside in the abdomen.
The large intestine rules the fluids, which have now caused fullness,
and is the place that is damaged by water qì.
Afterwards, the fluids are unable to ascend and reach the mouth and tongue,
causing dryness.
Three grams each of *jiāo mù, fáng jǐ, ting lì,* and *dá huáng,*
taken as a honey pill with each meal.

Commentary by Master Chéng[32] **程氏曰：**

防己、椒目導飲於前，大黃、葶藶推飲於後，前後分消則腹滿減而水飲行，脾氣轉而津液生矣。與上方互異處，當求其理。

Fáng jǐ and *jiāo mù* both guide rheum out through the front (urine), while *dà huáng* and *tíng lì* push rheum out through the back (bowels). Once separately eliminated through both ends, abdominal fullness is reduced and water-rheum moves. Subsequently, spleen qì is able to move and generate fluids. [One] must [clearly] seek out the reasoning and [thereby] distinguish the differences between this and the previous formula.

32. Most likely referring to Chéng Yúnlái 程雲來.

小半夏加茯苓湯

Xiǎo Bàn Xià Jiā Fú Líng Tāng

Minor Pinellia Decoction with Poria

治卒嘔吐，心下痞，膈間有水，眩悸者，主之。

A treatment for sudden vomiting and retching with glomus below the heart, which indicates water in the diaphragm, along with dizziness and palpitations, [this formula] rules it.

半夏（一升）生薑（半斤）茯苓（四兩）

bàn xià	半夏	200ml
shēng jiāng	生薑	24g
fú líng	茯苓	12g

上三味，以水七升，煮取一升五合，分溫再服。

Boil the three ingredients above in 1,400ml of water until reduced to 300ml. Divide and take warm in two doses.

Song 歌曰:

嘔吐悸眩痞又程，
四苓升夏八薑烹；
膈間有水金針度，
澹滲而辛得病情。

[When] vomiting, palpitations, dizziness, and glomus are all present,
cook twelve grams of *fú líng*, 200ml of *bàn xià*, and twenty-four grams of *shēng jiāng*.
The secret to treating water in the diaphragm
is to quietly percolate with acridity, [which] is suitable for the condition.

Commentary by [Chén] Yuánxī 男元犀按：

水滯於心下則為痞，水凌於心則眩悸，水阻胸膈，則陰陽升降之機不利，為嘔吐。方用半夏降逆，生薑利氣，茯苓導水，合之為滌痰定嘔之良方。

Stagnant water below the heart will cause glomus. Water intimidating the heart will cause dizziness and palpitations. Water obstructing the chest and diaphragm inhibits the upbearing and downbearing mechanism of yīn and yáng and causes vomiting. This formula uses *bàn xià* to downbear counterflow, *shēng jiāng* to disinhibit qì, and *fú líng* to guide water [downwards]. This combination is an effective prescription to flush out phlegm and stabilize vomiting.

五苓散
Wǔ Líng Sǎn
Five Substances Powder with Poria

歌見《傷寒》。

For the song, see the *Shāng Hán Lùn.*

治瘦人臍下有悸，吐涎沫而顛眩，此水也，此方主之。

A treatment for thin patients with palpitations below the umbilicus, vomiting of drool and spittle, withdrawal, and dizziness. This is water, [and] this formula rules it.

澤瀉（一兩一分）豬苓（三分，去皮）茯苓（三分）白朮（三分）桂（二分，去皮）[33]

zé xiè	澤瀉		3.75g
zhū líng	豬苓	skin removed	2.25g
fú líng	茯苓		2.25g
bái zhú	白朮		2.25g
guì [zhī]	桂［枝］	bark removed	1.5g

上五味，為末，白飲服方寸匕，日三服，多飲暖水，汗出愈。

Powder the five ingredients above, and take one gram with a white beverage,[34] three times daily. In addition, drink extra amounts of warm water, and once sweating is attained, recovery will ensue.

33. The dosage for the formula is open for debate, as some commentators and translators have chosen to use parts when discussing the measurement *fēn* (分), where the dosage for *zé xiè* is written as 1 *liǎng* (兩) and 1 part. However, the medicinals in the *Shāng Hán Lùn* version of *Wǔ Líng Sǎn* are measured in *liǎng* and *zhū* (銖). Where 1 *zhū* is the equivalent of 1/24 of a *liǎng* and according to this translation of the *Jīn Guì Fāng Gē Kuò* a *fēn* is the equivalent of 0.75g, it seems only fitting then, that the dosage of *zé xiè* should be 3.75g (1 *liǎng* and 1 *fēn*), and that the other medicinals be measured as 1 *fēn* = 0.75g.

34. White beverage: rice decoction or gruel.

Quotation by Yù Jiāyán 喻嘉言云:

水飲下鬱於陰中，挾其陰邪，鼓動於臍則為悸，上入於胃則吐涎沫，及其鬱極乃發，直上頭目，為顛為眩。五苓散利水以發汗，為分利表裏陰陽之法。

Water-rheum descends and is depressed within yīn. Complications by yīn evil agitate the umbilicus and cause palpitations. This [evil] ascends and enters the stomach, causing vomiting of drool and spittle, as well as the emergence of extreme depression. With ascension directly into the head and eyes, this results in withdrawal and dizziness. ***Wǔ Líng Sǎn*** disinhibits water, and promotes sweating, and is a method which separately disinhibits the exterior, interior, yīn and yáng.

Commentary by [Chén] Yuánxī 男元犀按:

臍下动氣，去朮加桂，仲師理中丸法也。茲何以臍下悸而用白朮乎？不知吐涎沫是水氣盛，必得苦燥之白朮方能制水；顛眩是土中濕氣化為陰霾上彌清竅，必得溫燥之白朮方能勝濕。證有兼見，法須變通。

With stirring qì below the umbilicus, remove *bái zhú* and add *guì zhī*. This is the method of Master Zhòng's *Lǐ Zhōng Wán*. Now here, why are we using *bái zhú* with palpitations below the umbilicus? [For those who] are unaware, vomiting of drool and spittle [is] due to the overabundance of water qì, [and therefore] a bitter drying *bái zhú* formula must be used to restrain water. Dizziness is due to damp qì within the earth transforming into a haze, which ascends and fills the clear orifices; [so therefore] we must use the warm and drying nature of *bái zhú* to overcome dampness. Because two patterns are simultaneously seen, we must be flexible with our methods.

附方
Fù Fāng
Attached Formulas

《外臺》茯苓飲
Wài Tái Fú Líng Yǐn
Poria Beverage from the *Wài Tái Mì Yào*

治心胸中有停痰宿水，自吐出水後，心胸間虛，氣滿不能食，消痰氣，令能食。

A treatment for collected phlegm and abiding water in the heart and chest with a vacuity of the heart and chest, fullness of qì, and an inability to eat following the spontaneous vomiting of water. [This formula] disperses phlegm-qì, and enables one to eat.

茯苓人參白朮（各三兩）枳實（二兩）橘皮（二兩半）生薑（四兩）

fú líng	茯苓	9g
rén shēn	人參	9g
bái zhú	白朮	9g
zhǐ shí	枳實	6g
jú pí	橘皮	7.5g
shēng jiāng	生薑	12g

上六味，以水六升，煮取一升八合，分溫三服，如人行八九裏，通作一服進之。

Simmer the six ingredients above in 1,200ml of water until reduced to 360ml. Divide and take warm in three doses, with an interval equal to the time it takes for an eight- or nine-*lǐ*[35] walk.

35. A *lǐ* is just shy of a mile or slightly more than half a kilometer.

Song 歌曰:

中虛不運聚成痰,
枳二兩參苓朮各三,
薑四橘皮二兩半,
補虛消滿此中探。

Central vacuity is unable to transport gatherings, which become phlegm.
Six grams of *zhǐ shí*, and nine grams each of *rén shēn, fú líng*, and *bái zhú*.
Twelve of *shēng jiāng*, and seven-and-a-half of *jú pí*,
[will] seek out the center by means of supplementing vacuity and dispersing fullness.

Commentary by [Chén] Yuánxī 男元犀按:

人參乃水飲症之大忌, 此方反用之, 蓋因自吐出水後虛氣作滿, 脾弱不運而設也。方中人參補脾氣, 白朮健胃氣, 生薑溫中散寒氣, 茯苓降水氣, 橘皮、枳實化痰運參朮, 徐徐斡旋於中, 以成其補虛消食散滿之妙用。此方施於病後調養則可, 若痰飲未散者, 切不可用。

Rén shēn is majorly contraindicated in water-rheum conditions, but is used in this formula, the reason being that following the spontaneous vomiting of water, fullness is caused by vacuous qì and spleen weakness failing to transport, [and therefore, this condition] is established. Within the formula, *rén shēn* is used to supplement spleen qì, *bái zhú* is used to fortify stomach qì, *shēng jiāng* warms the center, and scatters cold qì, *fú líng* downbears water qì, and *jú pí* and *zhǐ shí* transform phlegm and gently mediate the center by transporting *rén shēn* and *bái zhú*. These functions make this a wonderful formula to supplement vacuity, disperse food [accumulations], and dissipate fullness. This formula may be continued after the disease [has resolved] in order to harmonize and nourish, but if phlegm-rheum has not yet dissipated, it should not be used.

十棗湯
Shí Zǎo Tāng
Ten Jujube Decoction

歌見《傷寒》。

For the song, see the *Shāng Hán Lùn*.

咳家其脈弦，為有水，此主之。

In patients with cough who present with a wiry pulse, [this] indicates water, [and] this [formula] rules it.

支飲家，咳煩，胸中痛者，不卒死，至一百日或一歲，宜此湯主之。

For propping-rheum patients with coughing, vexation, and pain in the chest, who do not suddenly die and survive for a hundred days or up to one year, it is suitable to treat them with this decoction, for it rules [this condition].

Commentary by Wèi[36] 男蔚按:

凡人將咳之頃，喉間似哽非哽，似痒非痒，若有若無者，皆飲氣乾之也。飲氣一乾，則咳嗽作矣。除癆傷、積損，脈極虛、極細者，別有治法。若咳而脈弦，皆爲水飲，皆宜十棗湯攻之。若診得弦者，畏不敢用，其飲動肺則咳，動心則煩，搏擊陽氣則胸痛，即到一百日一歲之久，亦以此方爲背城之借，然亦危矣。此言治法當如是也，非謂必用此方，以致敗名取怨。

Whenever [one may] have a tendency to cough, or [experience a sensation] in the throat of choking but doesn't choke, and a throat which may or may not be itchy, whether it is distinct or not, this is always [due to] the assault of phlegm-rheum. When there is assault by rheum qì, coughing occurs. [In cases of] consumption damage, accumulation injuries, or [in patients with] extremely

36. Chén Wèi or Chén Yuánbào 元豹 was Chén Xiūyuán's eldest child. There is very little information available about him, as most references to Chén's children merely discuss Chén Yuánxī.

vacuous or thin pulses, one must be extremely careful, [and use] other treatment methods. In coughing with a wiry pulse, all [cases] are due to water-rheum, and [in these cases], it is suitable to use *Shí Zǎo Tāng* to attack it. [Some] during examination, when finding a wiry pulse, dare not use [this formula]. [If] rheum stirs the lungs then [there is] cough, [if rheum] stirs the heart then [there is] vexation, and [if] the yáng and qì struggle with [each other] then [there is] chest pain. [If one] survives for 100 days or up to one year, which is nevertheless also dangerous, one should still use this formula for the purpose of fighting to the last ditch. These are the treatment methods discussed [in the text], and without saying that [one] must use this formula [not using the formula] will [result in] complaints and damage [to one's] reputation.

Quotation by Yù [Jiāyán] 喻云:

咳嗽必因於痰飲，而五飲之中，獨膈上支飲最為咳嗽根底。外邪入而合之固嗽，即無外邪。而支飲漬入肺中，自令人咳嗽不已，況支飲久蓄膈上，其下焦之氣逆衝而上者，尤易上下合邪也。夫以支飲之故，而令外邪可內，下邪可上，不去支飲，其咳終無愈期矣。去支飲，用十棗湯，不嫌其峻。豈但受病之初，即病蓄已久，亦不能舍此別求良法。

Coughing is almost always due to phlegm-rheum, and amongst the five [kinds] of rheum; only propping-rheum above the diaphragm is most [often] the root of coughing. [If] external evil enters [the body], and [brings forth] a stubborn cough, then there is an absence of exterior evil. [If] propping-rheum enters and soaks the lungs, this will cause a person to cough incessantly. Moreover, [if] propping-rheum amasses above the diaphragm for an extended period of time, then the qì of the lower burner surges counterflow and ascends, [and this] makes it particularly easy for the evil to combine in the upper and lower [body]. This occurs because propping-rheum can cause external evil to [enter] the interior, and evils in the lower [body] to ascend. If propping-rheum is not eliminated, then one would be unable to recover from coughing for extended periods of time. To eliminate propping-rheum, use *Shí Zǎo Tāng*, yet do not blame [the formula] for its [excessive] harshness. For neither at the onset of the disease [nor] if it has amassed for a long time, [would one] abandon this [formula] in search of another excellent method!

小青龍湯

Xiǎo Qīng Lóng Tāng

Minor Blue-Green Dragon Decoction

歌見《傷寒》。

For the song, see the *Shāng Hán Lùn*.

咳逆倚息不得臥，此方主之。

[When there is] coughing with counterflow and propped breathing with an inability to lie down, this decoction rules it.

Commentary by [Chén] Yuánxī 元犀按:

十棗湯專主內飲而不及外邪，此方散外邪，滌內飲，為內外合邪之的方也，以下五方，皆本此方為加減。

Shí Zǎo Tāng specifically governs the treatment of interior rheum without the presence of extreme external evil. This formula dissipates exterior evil, and flushes away interior rheum, to treat a combination of internal and external evils. The following five formulas are all modifications of this formula.

桂苓五味甘草湯

Guì Líng Wǔ Wèi Gān Cǎo Tāng

Cinnamon Bark, Poria, Schisandra, and Licorice Decoction

治青龍湯下已，多唾口燥，寸脈沉，尺脈微，手足厥逆，氣從少腹上衝胸咽，手足痹，其面翕熱如醉狀，因復下流陰股，小便難，時復冒者，與此湯，治其氣衝 。

A treatment for when after taking *Xiǎo Qīng Long Tāng* there is copious spittle, a dry mouth, a deep pulse at the inch opening, and a faint pulse at the cubit position. [In addition] there is reverse counterflow in the hands and feet, qì surging up from the lower abdomen to the chest and throat, impediment in the extremities, a red flushed face as if drunk, and because of repeated downpour into the groin, there is difficult urination, and periodically recurring muddledness. Give this decoction to treat the surging qì.

按：脈沉微，支厥痹，面如醉，氣衝時復冒，似少陰陰陽不交之症，學者可於臨症時參辨之則可。

Commentary: [When there is] a deep and faint pulse, propping [rheum] with reversal impediment, a face as if drunk, and qì surging with periodic muddledness, this resembles a pattern of non-interaction between the yīn and yáng of shàoyīn. When arriving at these patterns, students can compare and differentiate these principles.

桂枝茯苓（ 各四兩 ）五味（ 半升 ）甘草（ 三兩，炙 ）

guì zhī	桂枝		12g
fú líng	茯苓		12g
wǔ wèi [zǐ]	五味［子］		100ml
gān cǎo	甘草	honey-fried	9g

上四味，以水八升，煮取三升，去滓，分溫三服 。

Simmer the four ingredients above in 1,600ml of water until reduced to 600ml. Remove the dregs, divide, and take warm in three doses.

Song 歌曰:

青龍卻礙腎元虧，
腎元虧而誤服之，
則動衝任之火，
致變為已下諸證。
上逆下流又冒時；
氣從少腹上衝胸咽，
或面熱如醉，
或熱氣流於兩股，
或小便難而昏冒，
忽上忽下，在陽無主，
如電光之閃爍無定，
味用半升苓桂四，
甘三扶土鎮衝宜。

Xiǎo Qīng Lóng Tāng may cause [further] depletion to the original [qì] of the kidney.
Original kidney qì was debilitated, and [*Xiǎo Qīng Lóng Tāng*]
was erroneously administered.
This led to the stirring and surging of conception vessel fire,
which changed into one of the various patterns [which follow] administration.
Ascending counterflow with downpour, in addition to periodic muddledness,
qì surging upward from the lower abdomen into the chest,
or a red flushed face as if drunk,
or warm qì flowing into the groin,
or difficult urination, and clouded veiling,
which fluctuate sharply, are [the result] of yáng not ruling,
and are unpredictable like the flickering of lightning.
100ml of *wǔ wèi zǐ*, twelve grams of *fú líng* and *guì zhī*,
and nine grams of *gān cǎo* are suitable to support earth and settle the surging.

Commentary by [Chén] Yuánxī 男元犀按:

仲師五味子必與乾薑同用，獨此方不用者，以誤服青龍之後衝氣大動，取其靜以制動，故暫停不用也。尤云：苓、桂能抑衝氣使之下行，然逆氣非斂不降，故以五味之酸斂其氣，土厚則陰火自伏，故以甘草之甘補其中也。

Master [Zhàng] Zhōngjǐng's *wǔ wei zǐ* is always combined with *gān jiāng*, [however] in this formula [*gān jiāng*] is not used. Following the erroneous administration of *Xiǎo Qīng Lóng Tāng*, there is major stirring of surging qì. Take this [formula] to tranquilize in order to control the stirring, and once it stops, there is no need to [continue] taking it. Yóu Zàijīng says *fú líng* and *guì zhī* are able to control surging qì, allowing it to move downwards, and [if] counterflow qì fails to go down due to a lack of restraint, sour *wǔ wèi zǐ* is used to restrain it. [Once] earth is thickened, yīn fire conceals itself, and for this reason sweet *gān cǎo* is used to supplement earth.

桂苓五味甘草去桂加薑辛湯

Guì Líng Wǔ Wèi Gān Cǎo Qù Guì Jiā Jiāng Xīn Tāng

Cinnamon Twig, Poria, Schisandra, and Licorice Decoction
with removed Cinnamon Twig and added Dried Ginger, Asarum, and Pinellia

治服前藥衝氣即低，而反更咳、胸滿者，此湯主之。

A treatment following the ingestion of the previous medicinals, which have lowered the surging qì but now there is coughing, and chest fullness. This decoction rules.

茯苓（四兩）甘草乾薑辛（三兩）五味子（半升）

fú líng	茯苓	12g
gān cǎo	甘草	9g
gān jiāng	乾薑	9g
xì xīn	細辛	9g
wǔ wèi zǐ	五味子	100ml

上五味，以水八升，煮取三升，去滓，溫服半升，日三服。

Simmer the five ingredients above in 1,600ml of water, until reduced to 600ml. Remove the dregs, and take 100ml warm, three doses per day.

Song 歌曰:

衝氣低時得桂苓之力而低。
咳寒飲漬肺則咳滿
寒飲貯胸則滿頻，
前方去桂益薑辛；
兩次用桂而邪不服，
以桂能去陽分凝滯之寒，
不能驅臟腑沉匿之寒，
必得乾薑、細辛大辛大熱，
方能洩胸中之滿而止咳也。

桂苓五味甘草去桂加薑辛湯

薑辛三兩根據原法，
原法通微便出新。

When surging qì is lowered, **the lowering [is due] to the strength of *guì zhī* and *fú líng*,**
[there is] coughing cold-rheum soaks the lungs, resulting in coughing and fullness;
cold-rheum is stored in the chest resulting in frequent fullness.
[This is] the previous formula with *guì zhī* removed and *gān jiāng* and *xí xīn* added.
***Guì zhī* has been used twice [yet] evils have not been dealt with.**
[The reason is] that *guì zhī* is able to eliminate congealed
and stagnant cold from the yáng aspect,
but is unable to expel deep and hidden cold from the viscera and bowels.
For this, one must use the great heat and acridity of *gān jiāng* and *xì xīn*,
[and as a result] the formula is able to discharge fullness from the chest and stop coughing.
Gān jiāng, xì xīn each nine grams according to the [*Xiǎo Qīng Lóng Tāng*] method,
[for this] is a proficient new advancement of the original method.

苓甘五味薑辛半夏湯

Líng Gān Wǔ Wèi Jiāng Xīn Bàn Xià Tāng

Poria, Licorice, Schisandra, Ginger, Asarum, and Pinellia Decoction

治服前藥咳滿即止，而更復渴，衝氣復發者，以細辛、乾薑為熱藥也。服之當遂渴，而渴反止者，為支飲也。支飲者，法當冒，冒者必嘔，嘔者復內半夏，以去其水。

A treatment **following the ingestion of the previous medicinals**, which have stopped the coughing and chest fullness, but thirst and surging qì have returned. This is because *xì xīn* and *gān jiāng* are hot-natured medicinals. After taking those medicinals, one should feel thirsty, but if the thirst is gone, this is due to propping-rheum. Propping-rheum typically causes dizziness, and this dizziness should cause vomiting. For vomiting, add *bān xiā* to eliminate water.

茯苓（四兩）甘草細辛乾薑（各三兩）半夏五味（各半升）

fú líng	茯苓	12g
gān cǎo	甘草	9g
xì xīn	細辛	9g
gān jiāng	乾薑	9g
bàn xià	半夏	100ml
wǔ wèi [zǐ]	五味［子］	100ml

上六味，以水八升，煮取三升，去滓，溫服半升，日三服。

Simmer the six ingredients above in 1,600ml of water until reduced to 600ml. Remove the dregs, and take 100ml warm, three doses per day.

Song 歌曰:

咳滿平時咳滿之病，
得薑辛而除。渴又加，
旋而不渴飲餘邪，
渴者，以辛薑之熱動之也；

渴反止者，
有餘飲以制燥也。
飲去則渴，
飲來則不渴而冒嘔。
冒而必嘔半升夏，
增入前方效可夸 。

Coughing and fullness have been calmed, **in coughing and fullness diseases,**
***gān jiāng* and *xì xīn* are used to eliminate it,** and thirst has increased again;
[if there is] an absence of thirst not long after, [this is due to] the surplus of rheum evil.
Thirst is the result of stirring caused by the heat of *xì xīn* and *gān jiāng*;
[but when] thirst has on the contrary stopped,
[this is because] there is a surplus of rheum, which restrains the dryness.
When rheum is eliminated, there will be thirst,
and when rheum returns, there will be an absence of thirst with dizziness and vomiting.
With dizziness there will [also] be vomiting, [and] adding in 100ml of *bàn xià,*
[will] greatly increase the [previous formulas] overall effectiveness.

Commentary by [Chén] Yuánxī 男元犀按:

前言氣衝，是真陽上奔，必用桂、苓招納之；此言氣衝，是熱藥鼓之，只用半夏以降逆則愈。且冒而嘔，半夏為止嘔之神药也。一本去甘草，恐甘而助呕也。

In the previous lines [there is] surging of qì, which is [the result of] true yáng running upwards. *Guì zhī* and *fú líng* must be used to absorb it. In these lines there is surging qì, which was roused by [the use of] hot medicinals, and only *bàn xià* is used to downbear counterflow and bring forth recovery. Moreover, there is dizziness and vomiting, and *bàn xià* is a divine medicinal for stopping vomiting. Other editions remove *gān cǎo* out of fear that its sweetness will stir vomiting.

苓甘五味薑辛半夏杏仁湯

Líng Gān Wǔ Wèi Jiāng Xīn Bàn Xià Xìng Rén Tāng

Poria, Licorice, Schisandra, Ginger, Asarum, Pinellia, and Apricot Kernel Decoction

治服藥前水去嘔止，其人形腫者，肺氣不行也。加杏仁主之。其症應內麻黄，以其人遂痹，故不內之，若逆而內之者，必厥，所以然者，以其人血虛，麻黄發其陽故也。

A treatment **prior to taking the medicinals**, [when] water [has been] eliminated and vomiting has stopped, [and now] the patient has generalized swelling, **[this is due to] lung qì failing to move.** Adding *xìng rén* rules it. For this pattern, one would normally add *má huáng*, but since the patient presents with impediment, it is not added. If one acts against the condition and adds [*má huáng*], this will cause reversal, the reason being that the patient has blood vacuity, and *má huáng* will act to effuse yáng.

茯苓（四兩）甘草乾薑細辛（各三兩）五味半夏杏仁（各半升）

fú líng	茯苓	12g
gān cǎo	甘草	9g
gān jiāng	乾薑	9g
xì xīn	細辛	9g
wǔ wèi [zǐ]	五味[子]	100ml
bàn xià	半夏	100ml
xìng rén	杏仁	100ml

上七味，以水一斗，煮取三升，去滓，溫服半升，日三服。

Simmer the seven ingredients above in 2,000ml of water until reduced to 600ml. Remove the dregs, and take 100ml warm, three doses per day.

Song 歌曰:

咳輕嘔止腫新增，
面腫須知肺氣凝；
前劑杏加半升煮，
可知一味亦規繩 。

The coughing has lightened, and vomiting has stopped, [but] now swelling has increased.
When the face is swollen, we must know that lung qì is congealed.
[This is] the previous formula, with 100ml of *xìng rén* added;
[as we] know, this is the principle [behind the use] of this one medicinal.

Commentary by [Chén] Yuánxī 男元犀按:

形氣，肺也。肺主皮毛，為治節之官，形腫者，肺氣不行，凝聚不通故也。加杏仁者，取其苦洩辛開，內通肺氣，外散水氣。麻黃亦肺家之藥，何以不用？慮其發越陽氣而重傷津液也。

Form and qì [are ruled by] the lungs. The lungs rule the skin and [body] hair, and are the officials in charge of the management and regulation [of qì and water]. Generalized swelling is the result of lung qì failing to move, and [with] congealing [of qì] there is lack of free flow. By adding *xìng rén*, we are able to drain due to its bitterness and open with its acridity, thereby freeing lung qì internally, and dissipating water qì in the exterior. *Má huáng* is also a medicinal, which is part of the lung family, so why is it not used? The reason is that if yáng qì is diffused in vacuous patients, fluids could be seriously damaged.

苓甘五味薑辛夏杏大黃湯

Líng Gān Wǔ Wèi Jiāng Xīn Xià Xìng Dà Huáng Tāng

Poria, Licorice, Schisandra, Ginger, Asarum, Pinellia, Apricot Kernel, and Rhubarb Decoction

治面熱如醉，此為胃熱上衝熏其面，以前方加大黃以利之。

A treatment for facial flushing as if drunk, which is caused by stomach heat surging upward and fuming the face. This is the previous formula with the addition of *dà huáng* in order to disinhibit it.

茯苓（四兩）甘草乾薑細辛（各三兩）五味半夏杏仁（各半升）大黃（三兩）

fú líng	茯苓	12g
gān cǎo	甘草	9g
gān jiāng	乾薑	9g
xì xīn	細辛	9g
wǔ wèi [zǐ]	五味［子］	100ml
bàn xià	半夏	100ml
xìng rén	杏仁	100ml
dà huáng	大黃	9g

上八味，以水一斗，煮取三升，去滓，溫服半升，日三服。

Simmer the eight ingredients above in 2,000ml of water until reduced to 600ml. Remove the dregs, and take 100ml warm, three doses per day.

Song 歌曰:

面熱如醉火邪殃，
胃熱上衝熏其面。
前劑仍增三兩黃，
驅飲辛溫藥一派，
別能攻熱制陽光。

Facial flushing as if drunk is a calamity [due to] fire evil.
Stomach heat surges upwards and fumes the face.
To the previous formula, add nine grams *dà huáng*,
[for] the acrid, warm group of medicinals, which expel rheum,
are not able to attack heat and restrain the brightness of yáng.

Commentary by [Chén] Yuánxī 男元犀按：

與衝氣上逆、發熱如醉者不同，彼因下焦陰中之陽虛，此不過肺氣不利，滯於外而形腫，滯於內而胃熱，但以杏仁利其胸中之氣，大黃洩其胃中之熱，則病愈矣。

Surging qì ascending counterflow, with flushing as if drunk is not the same [as this pattern]. The previous one is caused by yáng vacuity within yīn in the lower burner, and this one is the result of lung qì failing to move, which stagnates in the exterior, causing generalized swelling and stagnation in the interior with stomach heat. *Xìng rén* disinhibits qì in the chest, and *dà huáng* discharges heat in the stomach, bringing forth resolution of the condition.

從咳逆倚息起至此，六方五變為結局，學者當留心細認 。

From coughing and counterflow with propped breathing to this [current pattern], this concludes the six formulas with the five modifications that are used to address them. Students must [learn to] carefully recognize [them].

Quotation by Xú Zhōngkě 徐忠可云：

已上數方，俱不去薑、辛，即面熱如醉亦不去，何也？蓋以二味最能洩滿止咳，凡飲邪未去，須以二味刻刻預防也。

[In several] of the previous formulas above, neither *gān jiāng* nor *xì xīn* were removed, but why is it that [here] with facial flushing as if drunk, they are still not removed? The reason is that these two medicinals are very effective at discharging fullness and stopping coughing [and since] rheum evil has yet to be eliminated precautions must be taken against it.

按：孫真人最得此秘，觀麥門冬湯、五味子湯、補肺湯可見。余於此湯，凡桑白皮、阿膠、天冬、麥冬、茯苓、龍骨、牡蠣之類，隨證加入，其效無比。

Commentary: The immortal Sūn[37] was the most superior in [utilizing] this secret, especially when looking from the perspective [of his modified versions of] *Mài Mén Dōng Tāng, Wǔ Wèi Zǐ Tāng,* and *Bǔ Fèi Tāng.*[38] When I use this formula, [even when] adding medicinals such as *sāng bái pí, ē jiāo, tiān dōng, mài dōng, fú líng, lóng gǔ, mǔ lì,* and others, in accordance with the pattern, the effect [of this formula] is [still] unparalleled.

37. Sūn Sīmiǎo 孫思邈.

38. In Sūn's *Qiān Jīn Yào Fāng* 《千金要方》(Essential Prescriptions Worth a Thousand in Gold), the above formulas all contain either *shēng* or *gān jiāng* and *xì xīn* either on their own or in combination. Please refer to the text for exact formula ingredients.

小半夏加茯苓湯
Xiǎo Bàn Xià Jiā Fú Líng Tāng
Lesser Pinellia Decoction plus Poria

見上。

See above.

先渴後嘔，為水停心下，此屬飲家，此湯主之。

First thirst followed by vomiting is due to water stoppage below the heart. This belongs to the rheum family, and this decoction rules it.

半夏（一升）生薑（半斤）茯苓（三兩[39]）一法四兩。

bàn xià	半夏	200ml
shēng jiāng	生薑	24g
fú líng	茯苓	9g

上三味，以水七升，煮取一升五合，分溫再服。

Simmer the three ingredients above in 1,400ml of water until reduced to 300ml. Divide and take warm in two doses.

[Chén Yuán] Xi's received teachings from [Chén Xiūyuán] in the Zhí Qū Tíng[40] 犀在直趨庭聞訓曰：

此一節與上文似不相屬，而不知先生治咳，著眼在"水飲"二字，故於完篇之後，隨口逗出，此言外之提撕也。今試暢發其義。蓋飲水邪也，其本起於足太陽、足少陰二經，以二經為水之專司也。然太陽之

39. Another edition uses 12g.

40. The exact location or meaning behind the reference to the *Zhí Qū Tíng* is unclear, but it most likely refers to a hall where Chén Yuánxī received teachings from his father Chén Xiūyuán.

水為表水，膚腠不宜水氣，以致壅塞而為飲，則以小青龍發之。發之不能盡者，當從太陽之裏而疏瀹[41]之，十棗湯是也。少陰之水為裏水，下焦有寒，不能制伏本水，以致逆行而為飲，則以真武湯鎮之。鎮之而不盡服者，當從少陰之表而化導之，苓桂朮甘湯是也。更進一步，從中土以提防之，從高原而利導之。熟則生巧，不能以楮墨[42]傳也。近時喜用滑套之方，以六安煎、金沸草湯居於青龍之上，濟生腎氣丸、七味地黃丸駕乎真武之前，大體不礙者，吾亦姑如其說，究竟不如先生之原方效如桴鼓也。

[Although] this section and the preceding one are similar, [they are] not likely interrelated, and if we are not clear as to whether the teacher treated cough, and we concentrate on the two characters "water-rheum," then after finishing this chapter we would speak thoughtlessly, and be fixed on the external meaning of these words. I will now try to smoothly elucidate this meaning. The origin of water-rheum evil is in the foot tàiyáng and foot shàoyīn channels, which are the two channels responsible for the management of water. Tàiyáng's water is exterior water. It is inappropriate [for there to be] water qì in the skin and interstices, and when qì becomes congested and blocked, [this will result in] rheum, and *Xiǎo Qīng Lóng Tāng* is used to effuse it. [If] effusion is unable to terminate it, then [one] must course and dredge tàiyáng's interior, and *Shí Zǎo Tāng* is then used. Shàoyīn water is interior water, and when there is cold in the lower burner it is unable to control the root of water, which causes counterflow movement and becomes rheum. *Zhēn Wǔ Tāng* is a suitable formula to settle it. [If] settling is unable to terminate it, then [one] must transform and guide [downwards] from the exterior of shàoyīn, with *Líng Guì Zhú Gān Tāng*. To take it even one step further, [we could say that one is] safeguarding from central earth, and disinhibiting and guiding [down] from the uppermost source. Skill is generated from familiarity and is unable to be transmitted [through] mulberry paper and ink.[43] In modern times [people] like using lubricating formulas like *Liù Ān Jiān* and *Jīn Fèi Cǎo Tāng* as opposed to *Xiǎo Qīng Lóng Tāng*, and [formulas like] *Jì Shēng Shèn Qì Wán*, and *Qī Wèi Dì Huáng Wán*, before [utilizing] *Zhēn Wǔ Tāng*. In general, if one [cannot resist in following this way and] does not create [further] trouble, [then] I [can] comply with these words. [However] the results will be inferior to the masters' original formula whose effect is like [the sound from] sticks on a drum.

41. This character is the modern equivalent of *shū dǎo* 疏導 which means to dredge, or open up and clear obstructions.

42. The meaning of the character *chǔ* 墨 here is paper and ink, which refers to the written language or painting and calligraphy.

43. Mulberry paper and ink here refers to written work. My understanding of this passage is that Chén Yuánxi is saying that one needs to become familiar with the patterns they are presented with face to face, which is ultimately the best way to refine ones skill, as opposed to simply just learning through written work.

消渴小便不利淋病方

Xiāo Kě Xiǎo Biàn Bù Lì Lín Bìng Fāng

Formulas for Dispersion Thirst, Inhibited Urination, and Strangury Diseases

腎氣丸

Shèn Qì Wán

Kidney Qì Pill[44]

歌見婦人雜病 。

For the song, see [the section on] "Miscellaneous Gynecological Diseases."

治男子消渴，小便反多，以飲一斗，小便亦一斗，此丸主之 。

A treatment for men with dispersion thirst, that on the contrary urinate profusely, for when [they] drink 2,000ml of water, [they] urinate 2,000ml of water. This pill rules it.

Quotation by Yóu Zàijīng 尤在涇云：

水液屬陰，非氣不至，氣雖屬陽，中實含水，水與氣非一亦非二也。方中若無桂、附，何以振作腎中頹落之陽，游溢精氣，上輸脾肺邪？

Water belongs to yīn, [but] without qì, it fails to move. Although qì belongs to yáng, at its center it actually contains water, [for] water and qì are not different, nor the same. If there were no *guí zhī* or *fù zǐ* within the formula, how could it exert its effect on the kidneys, [prevent] yáng from declining, essential qì from wandering and spilling over, [and prevent the] transporting of evil upwards into the spleen and lungs?

44. For the formula, see above.

五苓散

Wǔ Líng Sǎn

Five-Substances Powder with Poria

歌見上。

For the song, see above.

治脈浮，小便不利，微熱消渴者，宜利小便發汗。

When treating a floating pulse, inhibited urination, and slight heat with dispersion thirst, it is suitable to disinhibit urination and promote sweating.

又治渴欲飲水，水入則吐者，名曰水逆。

In addition, [this formula treats] thirst with a desire to drink water, where upon ingestion of water, [the patient] vomits. This is called water counterflow.

Quotation by Yóu Zàijīng 尤在涇云:

熱渴飲水，水入不能已其熱，熱亦不能消其水，水與熱結，熱浮水外，故小便不利，微熱消渴。此利其與熱俱結之水，去其水外浮溢之熱，熱除水去，渴當自止。又熱已消而水不行，則逆而成嘔，及消渴之變證，曰水逆亦主之。

[When there is] heat and thirst [with a desire] to drink water, the water is ingested and is unable to stop the heat, and heat is also unable to disperse water. Water and heat bind, and heat floats [the] water to the surface, therefore there is inhibited urination, and slight heat with dispersion thirst. This [formula] disinhibits the water [which has] bound with heat, and removes the heat, which has floated and spilled over onto the surface of water. [Once both] heat and water are eliminated, thirst will stop on its own. In addition, if heat has already been dispersed, and water does not move, there will be counterflow, which will cause a transmutated pattern with vomiting and dispersion thirst, for which it is also said that [this formula] rules water counterflow.

文蛤散

Wén Gé Sǎn

Clamshell Powder

歌見《傷寒》。

For the song, see the *Shāng Hán Lùn.*

治渴欲飲水不止者，此散主之。

A treatment for thirst with an incessant desire to drink water, this powder rules it.

文蛤（五兩）

wén gé 文蛤 15g

上一味，杵為散，以沸湯五合，和服方寸匕。

Process the *wén gé* by pestling into a powder, and mix into 100ml of boiling water. Take one gram per dose.

Commentary by [Chén] Yuánxī 男元犀按：

與傷寒論文蛤散症不同。《傷寒論》云：肉上粟起，反不渴者，水寒浸肺，涌於外，遏於上，其熱被卻不得出也。文蛤入肺降肺氣，除濕熱，利小便，取其以殼治殼之義也。本節云渴欲飲水不止者，上無水濕遏鬱，中有燥熱上焚，脾乾胃燥，不能生津滋渴，飲水不止者，燥甚也。水性輕和，不能生津潤燥，文蛤則味咸寒，能育陰潤燥，洒除熱氣，下出小便，燥熱除，陰液長，而渴飲平矣。

This *Wén Gé Sǎn* pattern is not the same as that which is discussed in the *Shāng Hán Lùn.* It is said in the *Shāng Hán Lùn,* "[there will be] millet papules on the skin, with an absence of actual thirst" [which is the result of] cold water soaking the lungs, gushing into the exterior, and obstructing the upper, where it covers heat and prevents it from being eliminated. *Wén gé* enters the lung, downbears lung qì, eliminates damp-heat, and disinhibits urination. Here a strategy of using a shell to treat the shell[45] is utilized. In this section, it says thirst with incessant drinking of water. This is due to the obstruction and depression of water-damp in the upper burner, dryness-heat in the center setting fire to the upper, and spleen and stomach dryness being unable to engender fluids and quench thirst; therefore this incessant drinking of water is the result of severe dryness. The nature of water is light and harmonious, [but when] there is an inability to engender fluids and moisten dryness, the salty flavor and cold nature of *wén gé* is able to nourish yīn, moisten dryness, and eliminate heat qì, by descending outwards through urination, thereby eliminating dryness-heat, promoting the growth of yīn, and alleviating thirst.

45. I.e. the exterior.

栝蔞瞿麥丸

Guā Lóu Qú Mài Wán

Trichosanthes and Dianthus Pill

治小便不利者，有水氣，其人若渴者，宜之。

A treatment for inhibited urination, which indicates water qì, and if the patient is thirsty, [this formula] rules it.

薯蕷茯苓（各三兩）栝蔞根（二兩）附子（一枚，炮）瞿麥（一兩）

shǔ yù	薯蕷		9g
fú líng	茯苓		9g
guā lóu gēn	栝蔞根		6g
fù zǐ	附子	blast-fried	1 pc
qú mài	瞿麥		3g

上五味末之，煉蜜丸如梧子大，飲服二丸，日三服；不知，增至七八丸，以小便利，腹中溫為和。

Process the five ingredients above into a powder, and combine with refined honey to form pills the size of firmiana seeds. Take two pills, three times daily. If there is no effect, increase to seven or eight pills, and continue until the urination is uninhibited, and the abdomen is warm.

Song 歌曰:

小便不利渴斯成，
水氣留中液不生，
下焦火衰，中焦土弱，
水氣存於中，
阻其上下之津液不行。
三兩蕷苓瞿一兩，
一枚附子二蔞行。

[When] urination is inhibited, thirst is formed.
Water qì is retained in the center, and [yīn] fluids are not engendered.
[Here there is] decline of fire in the lower burner and central burner earth weakness.
The presence of water qì in the center
obstructs the movement of fluids in the upper and lower [burners].
Movement will occur with nine grams each of *shǔ yù* and *fú líng*, three grams *qú mài*,
a piece of *fù zǐ*, and six grams *guā lóu gēn*.

Commentary by [Chén] Yuánxī 男元犀按：

《內經》云：膀胱者，州都之官，津液存焉，氣化則能出矣。餘於氣化能出之義，而借觀之燒酒法，益恍然悟矣。酒由氣化，端賴鍋下之火力，方中附子補下焦之火，即其義也；酒釀成之水谷，收於鍋內而蒸之，其器具亦須完固，方中茯苓、薯蕷補中焦之土，即其義也；鍋下雖要加薪，而其上亦要頻換涼水，取涼水之氣，助其清肅以下行，則源源不竭，方中栝蔞根清上焦之力，即其義也；至於出酒之竅道，雖云未所當後，亦須去其積垢而通達，方中瞿麥一味專通水道，清其源而並治其流也，方後自注"腹中溫"三字，大有深義。

The *Huáng Dì Nèi Jīng* says the bladder is the regional rectifier, which stores fluids. These fluids are discharged through qì transformation. [In order] to understand the meaning behind discharge through qì transformation, [we] can use the methods [of producing] *shāo jiǔ*[46] [as an example], which should increase our realization in a flash! Alcohol is produced through qì transformation, which ultimately depends on the strength of fire at the bottom of the cauldron. Within the formula, the significance of *fù zǐ* is to supplement the fire of the lower burner. Alcohol is formed by the fermentation of water and grains, which have been gathered and steamed within the cauldron. As this vessel must also be firm and consolidated, the significance of *fú líng* and *shǔ yù* within the formula are to supplement the earth of the central burner. Although it is important to add firewood below the cauldron, [it is] also important [that] cool water is converted up top, so by applying the qì of cool water [we can] assist with depuration in order to move downwards, resulting in its' steady flow. The formula uses *guā lóu gēn* to clear the force of the upper burner, and thus the significance [of this medicinal] is to [apply the qì of cool water]. [Now] arriving at the opening from which the alcohol is discharged; while [in the case of alcohol distillation] it is said that there should not be [anything but clear alcohol] coming out the back. One must also eliminate the filth and facilitate free unimpeded flow. [Similarly] within the formula, *qú mài* is a specific medicinal [used] to free the waterways, clear [the] source [of the urination] and simultaneously manage its flow. After taking the formula [there is] spontaneous flow[47] and the abdomen will be warm. These last three characters have a very profound significance!

46. Famous *Táng* Dynasty wine.
47. Uninhibited urination.

蒲灰散

Pú Huī Sǎn

Typha Pollen Powder

小便不利者，此散主之；滑石白魚散、茯苓戎鹽湯並主之。

For inhibited urination, this powder rules it. *Huá Shí Bái Yú Sǎn* and *Fú Líng Róng Yán Tāng* are also indicated.

蒲灰（半分）[48]滑石（三分）

pú huī	蒲灰	½ part
huá shí	滑石	3 parts

上二味杵為散，飲服方寸匕，日三服。

Process the two ingredients above by pestling them into a powder, and take one gram in fluid, three doses per day.

Song 歌曰:

小便不利用蒲灰，
平淡無奇理備該；
半分蒲灰三分滑，
能除濕熱莫疑猜。

With inhibited urination, use *pú huī*.
There is nothing special nor strange to this logic;
for one should not be suspicious that
half a part of *pú huī* and three parts *huá shí*
can eliminate damp-heat.

48. The dosage of *pú huī* in the *Jīn Guì Yào Lüè* is seven parts. It is unclear as to the reason behind the drastic change in the present text.

滑石白魚散
Huá Shí Bái Yú Sǎn
Talcum and Lepisma Powder

滑石亂發（燒）白魚（各二分）

huá shí	滑石		2 parts
luàn fà	亂發	burnt	2 parts
bái yú	白魚		2 parts

上三味杵為散，飲服方寸匕，日三服。

Process the three ingredients above by pestling them into a powder. Take one gram with fluids, three doses per day.

Song 歌曰:

滑石餘灰亂發用火燒，
名血餘炭。與白魚，
專司血分莫躊躇，
藥皆平等擂調飲，
水自長流不用疏。

Huá shí and *yú huī*, ***luàn fà*** **is used, baked in fire,**
which is then called ***xuè yú tàn***, combined with *bái yú*
specifically [to enter] the blood aspect, [so] do not hesitate to use [them].
Pound equal parts of the medicinals and drink.
Water will spontaneously increase and flow, [and there is no need to] use a coursing [method].

茯苓戎鹽湯
Fú Líng Róng Yán Tāng
Poria and Halite Decoction

茯苓（ 半斤 ）白朮（ 二兩 ）戎鹽（ 彈丸大一枚 ）

fú líng	茯苓	24g
bái zhú	白朮	6g
róng yán	戎鹽	1 pc the size of a pellet

上三味，先將茯苓、白朮煎成，入戎鹽再煎，分溫三服。

After decocting the *fú líng* and *bái zhú*, add the *róng yán* and decoct again. Divide, and take warm in three doses.

Song 歌曰:

一枚彈大取戎鹽，
茯苓半斤火自潛，
更有白朮二兩佐，
源流不滯自濡沾。

One pellet-sized piece of *róng yán*
with twenty-four grams of *fú líng* and fire will spontaneously subdue;
furthermore, [with] six grams of the assistant *bái zhú*
the source and direction of flow will fail to stagnate and freely moisten.

Quotation by Yóu Zàijīng 尤在涇云:

蒲，香蒲也。寧原云：香蒲去濕熱，利小便，合滑石為清利小便之正法也。《別錄》云：白魚開胃下氣，去水氣，血餘療轉胞，小便不通，合滑石為滋陰益氣，以利其小便者也。《綱目》：戎鹽即青鹽，咸寒入腎，以潤下之性而就滲利之職，為驅除陰分水濕之法也。仲師不詳見證，而並出三方，以聽人之隨證審用，殆所謂引而不發者歟。

Pú is *xiāng pú*. Níng Yuán[49] says: *xiāng pú* eliminates damp-heat, and disinhibits urination. Combined with *huá shí* it is a standard treatment method for clearing and disinibiting the urine. The *Bié Lù*[50] says: *bái yú* opens the stomach, descends qì, eliminates [both] water qì and surplus of blood and treats a shifted bladder with urinary stoppage. Combine with *huá shí*, to enrich yīn, boost qì, and disinhibit urination. The *Gāng Mù*[51] says: *róng yán* is *qīng yán*, which is cold and enters the kidneys and by its nature of moist precipitation, is able to fulfill its duty in the function of percolating and disinhibiting, thereby expelling water-dampness from the yīn aspect. Master Zhòng[jǐng] was not very clear when presenting this pattern, as well as these three formulas, but [they] can [all] be used carefully when obeying and working in conjunction with a person's pattern, for this is what is referred to as simply "pulling the bow without shooting."[52]

按：蒲灰散主濕熱氣分，滑石白魚散主血分，茯苓戎鹽湯入腎除陰火。二散可療外瘡，多效。

Commentary: *Pú Huī Săn* rules damp-heat in the qì aspect; *Huá Shí Bái Yú Săn* rules the blood aspect; and *Fú Líng Róng Yán Tāng* enters the kidneys and eliminates yīn fire. Both powders are highly effective at treating external sores.

49. A *Míng* Dynasty physician (1522–1566) known for his work with food therapy, which he compiled into the *Shí Jiàn Běn Căo*《食鑑本草》(Examples of Food from the *Běn Căo*).

50. An alternate name for the *Míng Yī Bié Lù*《名醫別錄》(Specific Recordings by Famous Physicians) written by Táo Hóngjǐng 陶弘景 (456–536).

51. *Shén Nóng Běn Căo Jīng*《神農本草經》Anonymous.

52. Pulling the bow without shooting 引而不發 is an old Mèng Zǐ (Mencius) quote used to teach students proper form in archery. It is also used as a metaphor to help students be adequately prepared for understanding opportune times of action.

白虎加人參湯

Bái Hǔ Jiā Rén Shēn Tāng

White Tiger Decoction plus Ginseng

歌見《傷寒》。

For the song, see the *Shāng Hán Lùn.*

治渴欲飲水，口乾燥者，主之。

A treatment for thirst with a desire to drink water, and a dry and parched mouth, [this formula] rules it.

知母（六兩）石膏（一斤，碎）甘草（二兩）粳米（六合）人參（三兩）

zhī mǔ	知母		18g
shí gāo	石膏	smashed	48g
gān cǎo	甘草		6g
jīng mǐ	粳米		120ml
rén shēn	人參		9g

上五味，以水一斗，煮米熟，湯成，去滓，溫服一升，日三服。

Simmer the five ingredients above in 2,000ml of water until the rice [*jīng mǐ*] is cooked and the decoction is done. Remove the dregs and take 200ml warm, three doses per day.

Commentary by [Chén] Yuánxī 男元犀按：

小便不利者，水病也。天水一氣，金為水母，金氣不行，則水道不通。曰渴欲飲水，口乾燥者，火甚爍金，水源皆竭也。治求其本，故用白虎加人參湯潤燥金，補水源，使天氣降而水氣行，則渴燥自止矣。

Inhibited urination is a water disease. Both heaven and water are qì; metal is the mother of water, and when metal qì fails to move, there will be stoppage along the waterways. [In this line] it says that [there is] thirst with a desire to drink water, and a dry and parched mouth, which is the result of severe fire scorching metal, and exhausting the source of water. Treatment should seek out the root, therefore ***Bái Hǔ Jiā Rén Shēn Tāng*** should be used to moisten dry metal, and supplement the water source, to cause heavenly qì to downbear and move water qì, and afterwards thirst and dryness will spontaneously cease.

豬苓湯

Zhū Líng Tāng

Polyporus Decoction

歌見《傷寒》。

For the song, see the *Shāng Hán Lùn.*

治脈浮，發熱，渴欲飲水，小便不利者，宜之。

A treatment for a floating pulse, heat effusion, thirst with a desire to drink water, and inhibited urination, [this formula] is suitable.

豬苓（去皮）茯苓阿膠滑石澤瀉（各一兩）

zhū ling	豬苓	skin removed	3g
fú líng	茯苓		3g
ē jiāo	阿膠		3g
huá shí	滑石		3g
zé xiè	澤瀉		3g

上五味，以水四升，先煮四味，取二升，去滓，內膠烊消，溫服七合，日三服。

Simmer the four ingredients above [except for the *ē jiāo*] in 800ml of water until reduced to 400ml, remove the dregs, and dissolve the *ē jiāo* in the decoction. Take 140ml warm, three doses per day.

Commentary by [Chén] Yuánxī 男元犀按：

此與五苓散症迥別。五苓散主脾不轉輸而水停，故發汗利水，為兩解表裏法；此則胃熱甚而津液乾，故以清熱而滋燥，用育陰利水法，二者隻差一粟，學者自當細察焉。

This formula is quite different from ***Wǔ Líng Sǎn***. ***Wǔ Líng Sǎn*** [treats] failure of spleen transportation with collection of water. By promoting sweat and disinhibiting water, [***Wǔ Líng Sǎn***] achieves the dual function of resolving both the exterior and the interior. This [formula] treats severe stomach heat with dry fluids, using the method of clearing heat, enriching fluids, nourishing yīn and disinhibiting water. Students must carefully observe the subtle differences between these two [formulas].

水氣病方

Shuǐ Qì Bìng Fāng

Formulas for Water Qì Diseases

越婢加朮湯

Yuè Bì Jiā Zhú Tāng

Escape Restraint Decoction plus Ovate Atractylodes

即越婢湯加白朮四兩。方見下。

This is *Yuè Bì Tāng* with 12g of *bái zhú* added. See below for the formula.[53]

治裏水，一身面目黃腫，其脈沉，小便不利，故令病水。假令小便自利，此亡津液，故令渴，此湯主之。

A treatment for interior water with yellowing and swelling of the entire body, face and eyes, a deep pulse, and inhibited urination, which is referred to as water disease. When urination is naturally uninhibited, this results in fluid collapse, which causes thirst. This decoction rules it.

麻黃（六兩）石膏（半斤）生薑（三兩）甘草（二兩）白朮（四兩）大棗（十五枚）

má huáng	麻黃	18g
shí gāo	石膏	24g
shēng jiāng	生薑	9g
gān cǎo	甘草	6g
bái zhú	白朮	12g
dà zǎo	大棗	15 pcs

上六味，以水六升，先煮麻黃去上沫，內諸藥，煮取三升，分溫三服。惡風加附子一枚，炮。

53. In addition see *Qiān Jīn Yuè Bì Jiā Zhú Tāng*《千金》越婢加朮湯 in Volume 1, p.125.

Of the six ingredients above, first simmer the má huáng in 1,200ml of water. Remove the foam from the top, add all the other medicinals, and simmer until reduced to 600ml. Divide and take warm in three doses. For aversion to wind, add one piece of blast-fried *fù zǐ*.

Song 歌曰:

裹水脈沉面目黃，
水風相搏濕為殃；
專需越婢平風水，
四兩朮司去濕良 。

Interior water [with a] deep pulse, and yellowing of the face and eyes;
wind and water contend with each other [bringing forth] disaster
[in the form of] dampness. *Yuè Bì Tāng* is specifically needed to calm wind and water;
twelve grams *bái zhú* is excellent for managing the discharge of dampness.

Commentary by [Chén] Yuánxī 男元犀按:

水被熱蓄，氣為濕滯，致外不得通陽而作汗，內不能運氣而利水，故令病水。云：假令小便自利三句，疑非裏水病也。越婢湯發肌表之邪，以清內蓄之熱，加白朮運中土，除濕氣，利其小便，此分消表裏法也。或云：越婢散肌表之水，加白朮止渴生津也。

Water has amassed with heat, and qì is stagnant due to dampness. [As a result] there is an inability to sweat, due to the lack of free [flow] of yáng in the exterior, while in the interior, the inability of qì to move in order to disinhibit water, results in water disease. In the above three sentences where it says if urination is naturally uninhibited, [I] suspect [this] is not an interior water disease. *Yuè Bì Tāng* effuses evil from the fleshy exterior, and clears interior amassed heat. *Bái zhú* is added to move center earth, eliminate damp qì, and disinhibit the urination. This [formula] utilizes a strategy of separately dispersing both the exterior and interior. Some say that *Yuè Bì Tāng* dissipates water from the fleshy exterior, and by adding *bái zhú* thirst is alleviated and fluids are generated.

按：豈有小便自利亡津液而作渴者，仍用此湯，不顧慮其重傷津液乎？

Commentary: How can some still use this formula when the urination is uninhibited, and there is fluid collapse with thirst, without worrying about seriously damaging fluids?

防己黄芪湯

Fáng Jǐ Huáng Qí Tāng

Fáng Jǐ and Astragalus Decoction

歌見濕病中。

For the song, see [the section on] "Dampness Diseases."

治風水，脈浮身重，汗出惡風者，此湯主之。

A treatment for wind-water with a floating pulse, generalized heaviness, sweating, and aversion to wind. [This formula] rules it.

防己（一兩）甘草（半兩，炒）白朮（七錢半）黃芪（一兩一分，去蘆）

fáng jǐ	防己		3g
gān cǎo	甘草	honey-fried	1.5g
bái zhú	白朮		2.25g
huáng qí	黃芪	remove the non-medicinal parts	3.75g

上銼麻豆大，每服五錢匕，生薑四片，大棗一枚，水盞半，煎八分，去滓，溫服，良久再服。喘者加麻黃半兩，胃中不和者加芍藥三分，氣上衝加桂枝三分，下有陳寒者加細辛三分。服後當如蟲行皮中，從腰下如冰，後坐被上，又以一被繞腰以下，溫令微汗，差。

Grate the above ingredients to the size of *má dòu*. For each dose, take five *qían*-spoons full. With four pieces of *shēng jiāng* and one piece of *dà zǎo*, simmer [each dose] in half a cup of water [until reduced] to eight tenths. Remove the dregs and take warm. For panting, add one-and-a-half grams of *má huáng*. For disharmony in the stomach, add two-and-a-quarter grams of *sháo yào*. For upsurging qì, add two-and-a-quarter grams of *guì zhī*. For stale cold in the lower body, add two-and-a-quarter grams of *xì xīn*. After taking [this decoction], it will feel like bugs moving inside the skin and from the waist down like ice. Then have [the patient] sit on top of a blanket and wrap them in another blanket below the waist. Keep them warm to induce mild sweating, [and then there will be] recovery.

Commentary by [Chén] Yuánxī 男元犀按:

惡風者，風傷肌腠也。身重者，濕傷經絡也。脈浮者，病在表也。何以不用桂枝、麻黄以發表祛風，而用防己、黄芪以補虛行水乎？蓋以汗出為腠理之虛，身重為土虛濕勝。

Aversion to wind is due to wind damaging the interstices. Generalized heaviness [is due to] dampness damaging the channels and network vessels. A floating pulse [is due to] disease in the exterior. Why would one not use *guì zhī* or *má huáng* to effuse the exterior and eliminate wind, but instead use *fáng jǐ* and *huáng qí* to supplement vacuity and move water? This is because the sweating [here] is due to vacuity of the interstices, and the generalized heaviness is the result of vacuity of earth with the prevalence of dampness.

故用黄芪以走表塞空；棗、草、白朮以補土勝濕；生薑辛以去風，溫以行水，重用防己之走而不守者，領諸藥環轉於周身，使上行下出，外通內達，迅掃而無餘矣。

Therefore, use *huáng qí* to penetrate the exterior and fill up emptiness. [*Dà*] *zǎo*, [*gān*] *cǎo*, and *bái zhú* are used to supplement earth and prevail over dampness. *Shēng jiāng* eliminates wind with its acridity, and moves water with its warmth. A larger dose of *fáng jǐ* penetrates everywhere, thereby leading the other medicinals to circulate throughout the entire body. [By] causing upward movement and lower expulsion, [one] frees the outside and reaches the inside [resulting in] a rapid sweeping without any surplus.

越婢湯

Yuè Bì Tāng

Escape Restraint Decoction

治風水惡風，一身悉腫，脈浮不渴，續自汗出，無大熱，此湯主之。

A treatment for wind-water with an aversion to wind, generalized swelling, a floating pulse, an absence of thirst, periodic spontaneous sweating, and an absence of great heat; this decoction rules it.

麻黄（ 六兩 ）石膏（ 半斤 ）生薑（ 三兩 ）甘草（ 二兩 ）大棗（ 十二枚 ）

má huáng	麻黄	18g
shí gāo	石膏	24g
shēng jiāng	生薑	9g
gān cǎo	甘草	6g
dà zǎo	大棗	12 pcs

上五味，以水六升，先煮麻黄，去上沫，内諸藥，煮取三升，分溫三服，惡風加附子一枚；風水加朮四兩。

Use 1,200ml of water for the five ingredients above. First, boil the *má huáng*, removing the foam collecting on top, add the remaining ingredients, and boil until reduced to 600ml. Divide and take warm in three doses. If there is an aversion to wind, add one piece of *fù zǐ*, and with wind-water, add 12g of *bái zhú*.

Song 歌曰:

一身悉腫屬風多，
水為風翻涌巨波；
二草三薑十二棗，
石膏八兩六麻和。

Generalized heaviness is commonly due to wind,
for great waves are created when water is driven by wind;

this is harmonized with six grams of *gān cǎo,* nine of *shēng jiāng,* twelve pieces of *dà zǎo,* twenty-four grams of *shí gāo* and eighteen of *má huáng.*

Commentary by [Chén] Yuánxī 男元犀按:

惡風者，風也。一身悉腫者，水也。脈浮者，風發也，風為陽邪，風動則水火戰而浪涌矣，涌於上則不渴，涌於外則續自汗出。云無大熱者，熱被水蔽，不得外越，內已醞釀而成大熱矣。前章云身重，為濕多；此章云一身悉腫，為風多。風多氣多熱亦多，繫屬猛風，故君以石膏重鎮之品，能平息風浪以退熱，引麻黃直越其至陰之邪，協生薑散肌表之水，一物而兩握其要也。又以棗、草安中養正，不慮其過散傷液，所以圖萬全也。

Aversion to wind is [due to] wind. Generalized swelling is [due to] water. A floating pulse is [due to] to effusion of wind. Wind is a yáng evil, and when stirred, causes a struggle between water and fire [which results in] surging. [If there is an] upward surge, there [will be] a lack of thirst, and [if there is] a surge towards the exterior, there [will be] continuous spontaneous sweating. [In] this line, it is said, that there is an absence of great heat, [which is due to] heat being covered by water, and unable to thrust out externally. [Heat] has already been brewing internally and consequently becomes great heat. The previous line says "body heaviness" is the result of copious dampness. This line says, "generalized body swelling," which is due to copious wind. While wind is copious, so, too, are qì and heat, which have bound together to create a fierce wind. Therefore, the sovereign is *shí gāo,* which is a heavy settling substance that is able to calm and extinguish unrestrained wind in order to abate heat and guide *má huáng* to directly reach the yīn evil. [*Shí gāo*] assists *shēng jiāng* in dissipating water from the fleshy exterior. [This] one substance (*shí gāo*) holds two important keys (*má huáng* and *shēng jiāng*). Moreover, *dà zǎo,* and *gān cǎo* are able to calm the center, and nourish the right [qì], to keep one from worrying about excessive dissipation damaging fluids. Therefore, [this formula] covers every aspect.

防己茯苓湯
Fáng Jǐ Fú Líng Tāng
Stephania Root and Poria Decoction

治皮水四肢腫，水氣在皮膚中，四肢聶聶動者，此湯主之 。

A treatment for skin water [disease] with swelling of the four extremities, and water qì in the skin causing slight twitching of the four extremities; this decoction rules it.

防己黃芪桂枝（ 各三兩 ）茯苓（ 六兩 ）甘草（ 二兩 ）

fáng jǐ	防己	9g
huáng qí	黃芪	9g
guì zhī	桂枝	9g
fú líng	茯苓	18g
gān cǎo	甘草	6g

上五味，以水六升，煮取二升，分溫三服 。

Simmer the five ingredients above in 1,200ml of water until reduced to 400ml. Divide and take warm in three doses.

Song 歌曰:

四肢聶聶動無休，
皮水情形以此求；
己桂耆三草二兩，
茯苓六兩砥中流 。

In twitching of the four extremities without rest,
[a condition of] skin water is to blame;
the nine grams of *fáng jǐ, guì zhī,* and *huáng qí,* [with] six grams *gān cǎo,*
and eighteen of *fú líng,* play an indispensable role.

Quotation by Xú Zhōngkě 徐忠可云：

藥亦同防己黄芪湯，但去朮加桂、苓者，風水之濕在經絡近內，皮水之濕在皮膚近外，故但以苓協桂，滲周身之濕，而不以朮燥其中氣也。不用薑、棗者，濕不在上焦之營衛，無取乎宣之也。

[This formula contains] the same medicinals as *Fáng Jǐ Huáng Qí Tāng*, but with *bái zhú* removed, and *guì zhī* and *fú líng* added. The dampness of wind-water is in the channels and network vessels close to the interior, and the dampness of skin water is in the skin close to the exterior. Therefore, we only need *fú líng* to assist *guì zhī* in percolating dampness throughout the entire body, and there is no need to use *bái zhú* to dry center qì. Neither *shēng jiāng* or *dà zǎo* are used, as dampness is not in the construction or defense of the upper burner, and does not need to be diffused.

越婢加朮湯

Yuè Bì Jiā Zhú Tāng

Escape Restraint Decoction plus Ovate Atractylodes[54]

歌見上。

For the song, see above.

裏水病，此湯主之；甘草麻黄湯亦主之。

For interior water diseases, this decoction rules. *Gān Cǎo Má Huáng Tāng* also rules.[55]

Commentary by [Chén] Yuánxī 男元犀按:

風水，皮水之外，有正水而兼色黄，名裏水。裏水雖無發汗之法，而邪盛正不衰者，亦必藉麻黄之力深入其中，透出於外，以收捷效。今色黄是濕熱雜於內，宜此湯；如寒氣凝結於內，宜甘草麻黄湯。

Wind-water is skin water in the exterior. Regular water with concurrent yellowing is called interior water. Sweat promotion is not [typically] used in interior water [patterns]. However, since evils are exuberant and right qì is not debilitated, [we] may take advantage of *má huáng's* strength [and ability] to penetrate deeply to outthrust [evil] to the exterior, in order to achieve quick resolution. This yellowing is [the result of] dampness and heat mixing in the interior, and it is suitable [to administer] this decoction. If cold qì is congealed and bound in the interior, it is suitable to give *Gān Cǎo Má Huáng Tāng*.

---

54. For the formula, see above.

55. Some commentators believe that interior water here should actually be read as skin water, and have even gone so far as to change *lǐ shuǐ* 裏水 (interior water) into *pí shuǐ* 皮水 (skin water).

甘草麻黄湯
Gān Cǎo Má Huáng Tāng
Licorice and Ephedra Decoction

甘草（ 二兩 ）麻黃（ 四兩 ）

gān cǎo	甘草	6g
má huáng	麻黄	12g

上二味，水五升，先煮麻黃，去上沫，內甘草，煮取三升，溫服一升，重覆汗出，不汗，再服 。慎風寒 。

Use 1,000ml of water for the two ingredients above, first boiling the *má huáng*, removing the foam collecting on top, and then adding the *gān cǎo*. Boil until reduced to 600ml, and take 200ml warm. Cover up to promote a sweat, and if there is no sweating, take another dose. Avoid wind and cold.

Song 歌曰:

裏水原來自內生，
一身面目腫黃程；
甘須二兩麻黃四，
氣到二藥上宣肺氣，
中助土氣，外行水氣。
因知水自行 。

Interior water was originally generated from within the interior.
[There is] swelling and yellowing in the body, face and eyes,
[thus] six grams of *gān cǎo* is required along with twelve [grams] of *má huáng*.
When qì arrives, **[the] two medicinals will ascend and diffuse lung qì,**
assist earth qì, and move water in the exterior;
[it is] known that water will move on its own.

Commentary by [Chén] Wèi 男蔚按:

麻黄發汗最捷。徐靈胎謂其無氣無味，不專一經，而實無經不到。蓋以出入於空虛之地，凡有形之氣血，不得而御之也。

Má huáng is the quickest [medicinal] to promote sweating. Xū Língtāi said that [*má huáng*] is one without qì, flavor, or an affinity to a specific channel, [and] indeed reaches all channels. Since [*má huáng*] comes from empty space, all substantial qì and blood [would] be unable to handle it.

麻黃附子湯

Má Huáng Fù Zǐ Tāng

Ephedra and Aconite Decoction

歌見《傷寒》。

For the song, see the *Shāng Hán Lùn*.

麻黃（三兩）甘草（二兩）附子（一枚，炮）

má huáng	麻黃		9g
gān cǎo	甘草		6g
fù zǐ	附子	blast-fried	1 pc

上三味，以水七升，先煮麻黃，去上沫，內諸藥，煮取二升半，溫服八分，日三服。

Of the three ingredients above, first boil the *má huáng* in 1,400ml of water. Remove the foam collecting on the surface, toss in the various [other] medicinals, and simmer until reduced to 500ml. Take 160ml warm, three doses per day.

杏子湯

Xìng Zǐ Tāng

Apricot Kernel Decoction[56]

闕徐、尤云：疑是麻杏甘石湯。

[The formula] is lost. Xú Língtái, and Yóu Zàijīng had [both] doubted that this formula is *Má Xìng Gān Shí Tāng.*

水之為病，其脈沉小，屬少陰，浮者為風，無水虛脹者為氣。水，發其汗即已。脈沉者，宜麻黃附子湯；浮者，宜杏子湯。

In water disease, the pulse is deep and small, which belongs to shàoyīn. A floating pulse is due to wind, and the absence of water with vacuity distention, belongs to qì. [With] water [diseases in the exterior], promoting sweat will resolve it. When the pulse is deep, it is suitable to give *Má Huáng Fù Zǐ Tāng*; and when the pulse is floating, one can use *Xìng Zǐ Tāng.*

客問曰：《金匱》水氣篇杏子湯方闕，諸家注說疑為麻杏甘石湯，不知是否？犀答曰：非也。麻杏甘石湯，《傷寒論》治發汗後汗出而喘，主陽盛於內也。本節云：水之為病，發其汗即已。未云熱之為病自汗出也。蓋麻杏甘石湯治內蘊化熱自汗出之症，此水之為病，發其汗為宜。則麻杏甘石湯不可用矣。

The disciple asked: The formula *Xìng Zǐ Tāng* from the *Jīn Guì Yào Lüè* section on water qì [disease] is missing. All annotators say that they suspect [that this formula] is *Má Xìng Gān Shí Tāng*, and I do not know whether it is or is not. Xī responds: It is not. *Má Xìng Gān Shí Tāng* from the *Shāng Hán Lùn* treats sweating and panting following the promotion of sweat, and rules yáng exuberance in the interior. This section says: In water disease, the promotion of sweat will resolve it. It does not mention spontaneous sweating [caused by] heat. *Má Xìng Gān Shí Tāng* treats a pattern of spontaneous sweating due to heat brewing in the interior, and [the indication of] this [formula] is water disease where it is suitable to promote sweating, so therefore, *Má Xìng Gān Shí Tāng* cannot be used.

---

56. Throughout the years there have been numerous commentaries and discussions as to the actual ingredients of this formula. Several physicians have considered this formula to be *Má Xìng Shí Gān Tāng*. Others have thought it to be *Gān Cǎo Má Huáng Tāng* with *xìng zǐ*, while others suspect it to be *Má Xìng Yì Gān Tāng*. Since the actual ingredients were left out of Chén's original work, I have opted to leave them out as well.

客又曰：何以知杏子湯，方用麻黃而不用石膏乎？余答曰：師云：水病發其汗即已，故知其必用麻黃，而不用石膏矣。夫以石膏質重，寒涼之性能除裏熱，清肺胃，同麻黃、杏仁降逆鎮喘，外則旋轉於皮毛，用之退熱止汗則可，用之發表驅寒則不可耳。然則此篇師言脈沉小屬少陰，用附子溫經散寒，主石水之病，即可知脈浮屬太陽，用杏子啟太陰之氣，主正水之病，為變其脈症言之也。恐石膏之凝寒，大有關於脾腎，故不可用焉。

The disciple asks again: Why does *Xìng Zǐ Tāng* use *má huáng* and not *shí gāo*? My response: The master says that in water disease, promoting sweat will resolve it, therefore [from this] we know that *má huáng* should be used, and not *shí gāo*! *Shí gāo* is a heavy substance, and its cold nature is able to eliminate interior heat, and clear the lungs and stomach. Together, [with] *má huáng* and *xìng rén* [they can] downbear counterflow and settle panting. In the exterior they work on the skin and hair, [therefore] using [*shí gāo*] to abate heat and stop sweating is okay, while using [*shí gāo*] to effuse the exterior and expel cold is not! In this chapter the master says that the pulse is deep and small, which belongs to shàoyīn, so [therefore] *fù zǐ* is used to warm the channels and disperse cold, and [it] rules [the treatment of] stone water disease. Namely, [we] know that a floating pulse belongs to tàiyáng, and *xìng zǐ* is used to open the qì of tàiyīn, and rules regular water disease. Thus, these variances can be deciphered through the pulse signs. Due to fear of the congealing cold of *shí gāo*, which has a direct relationship to the spleen and kidneys, it cannot be used.

高明如徐忠可及二張二程，俱疑為麻杏甘石湯，甚矣！讀書之難也。而余以為其即麻黃、杏仁、甘草三味，不知是否？以俟後之學者，客悅而去。

Brilliant [physicians] like Xú Zhōngkě, as well as the two Zhāngs and two Chéngs,[57] all very much doubt that [this formula] is *Má Xìng Gān Shí Tāng*! This is difficult to read and understand! In addition, I believe that this formula is composed of *má huáng*, *xìng rén*, and *gān cǎo*, but I am not sure. The answer is left for future scholars [to determine]. The disciple was satisfied and left.

57. It is unclear which Chéngs he is referring to, but presumably one would be Chéng Yúnlái 程雲來. As for the Zhāngs, this could either be a reference to Zhāng Zhìcōng 張志聰 and Zhāng Lìngsháo 張令韶, or to Zhāng Shíwán 張石頑 and Zhāng Jǐngyuè 張景岳.

蒲灰散

Pú Huī Sǎn

Typha Pollen Powder[58]

歌見消渴 。

For the song, see [the section on] "Wasting Thirst."

治厥而為皮水者，此主之 。

For treating adverse skin water, this [formula] rules.[59]

Commentary 按:

皮水久而致潰，為逆而不順之證，以此散外敷之。此厥字言證之逆，非四肢厥逆之謂也。諸家多誤解。

Enduring skin water causing [skin] rupturing is an adverse and unfavorable pattern, [and is treated] by applying this powder to the exterior. [Here] the reversal character 厥 is describing an adverse pattern, and not the reversal counterflow associated with coldness of the four extremities. This is commonly misunderstood!

---

58. For the formula, see above.

59. Many commentators believe that this line should be read as reversal and skin water, which manifests with skin water and coldness of the extremities due to obstructed yáng in the chest being unable to reach and warm the extremities. However, as can be seen from Chén's commentary, he believed that this is incorrect and the line simply alludes to an adverse pattern of skin water.

黄芪芍藥桂枝苦酒湯

Huáng Qí Sháo Yào Guì Zhī Kǔ Jiǔ Tāng

Astragalus, Peony, Cinnamon Twig and Vinegar Decoction

治黄汗病，身體腫，發熱，汗出而渴，狀如風水，汗沾衣，色正黄如柏汁，脈自沉，從何得之？以汗出入水中浴，水從汗孔入得之，此湯主之。

A treatment for yellow sweat disease where there is generalized swelling, heat effusion, and sweating with thirst, which resembles wind-water. Sweat soaks through the clothing and has a deep-yellow color that resembles the juice of *huáng bái*, and the pulses are deep. From where does this condition arise? It arises when one takes a bath while sweating, [and] water enters through the pores. This decoction rules it.

黄芪（五兩）芍藥桂枝（各三兩）

huáng qí	黄芪	15g
sháo yào	芍藥	9g
guì zhī	桂枝	9g

上三味，以苦酒一升、水七升相合，煮取三升，溫服一升，當心煩，服至六、七日乃解。若心煩不止者，以苦酒故也。

Simmer the three ingredients above in 200ml of vinegar, combined with 1,400ml of water, until reduced to 600ml, and take 200ml warm. Heart vexation may be present, which should resolve after six or seven days. If the heart vexation fails to cease, then this is due to the vinegar.

Song 歌曰:

黄汗脈沉出汗黄，
水傷心火鬱成殃；
師云：汗出入水中浴，
水氣從汗孔入而傷其心，
故水火相浸而色黄，
水氣搏結而脈沉也。

黃芪五兩推方主，
桂芍均三苦酒勷。
止汗太急，故心煩也，
至六、七日乃解者，
正復而邪自退也。

In yellow sweating [disease] the pulse is deep, and [there is the] issuing of yellow sweat.
Water damages heart fire, which depresses and brings forth disaster.
The master said: [if one] sweats while bathing,
water qì will enter through the pores and damage the heart.
Water and fire will immerse in one another and cause yellowing.
Water and qì contend and bind, and the pulse will be deep.
Fifteen grams of *huáng qí* is praised as the ruler of the formula,
guì zhī and *sháo yào* both at nine grams are assisted by the vinegar.
If sweat is stopped too urgently, this will result in heart vexation.
This should resolve after six or seven days,
when the right [qì] is restored and the evil has abated on its own.

Commentary by [Chén] Yuánxī 男元犀按:

桂枝行陽，芍藥益陰，黃芪氣味輕清，外皮最厚，故其達於皮膚最捷，今煮以苦酒，則直协苦酒之酸以止汗，但汗出於心，止之太急，反見心煩，至六七日，正復邪退，煩必自止。而不止者，以苦酒阻其餘邪未尽故也。

Guì zhī moves yáng and *sháo yào* boosts yīn. The qì and flavor of *huáng qí* is light and clear, with the outer skin being the richest, therefore, it can reach the skin quite swiftly. Nowadays, this [decoction] is boiled with vinegar, for the sour taste of the vinegar can directly assist in stopping sweating. However, sweat issues from the heart, and since it was stopped too quickly, on the contrary we see heart vexation. After six or seven days, once the right [qì] has been restored and evil has abated, the vexation should stop on its own. But since it has not stopped, this is due to the vinegar, which has obstructed the elimination of the remaining evil.

Additional Commentary 又按:

凡看書宜活看，此证亦有从酒後汗出當风所致者，虽有外水，而所出之汗，是亦水也。凡脾胃受湿，湿久生热，湿热交蒸而成黄，皆可以汗出入水浴之意悟之也。

Whenever reading [other] texts [one] must [always] be flexible. This pattern is also caused by wind when there is sweating following [the ingestion] of alcohol. Although there is water on the surface, [there is] the emission of sweat, which is also water. Whenever the spleen and stomach suffer from dampness, and [are] left for long periods of time, dampness will generate heat. Dampness and heat will interact, steam, and cause yellowing, thus [one] can understand the significance behind sweating while bathing.

桂枝加黄芪湯

Guì Zhī Jiā Huáng Qí Tāng

Cinnamon Twig Decoction plus Astragalus

黄汗之病，兩脛自冷；假令發熱，此屬歷節 。食已汗出，又身常暮盜汗出者，此榮氣也 。若汗出已，反發熱者，久久其身必甲錯；發熱不止者，必生惡瘡，若身重，汗出已輒輕者，久久必身瞤，瞤即胸中痛，又從腰以上汗出，下無汗，腰髖弛痛，如有物在皮中之狀，劇者不能食，身疼痛，煩躁，小便不利，此為黄汗，桂枝加黄芪湯主之 。

Diseases of yellow sweat typically manifest with spontaneous cold of [the] lower legs. If there is heat effusion, this is due to joint running [disease]. With sweating after eating, and frequent sweating in the evening, this is taxation qì.[60] If heat effusion occurs after one has sweat, encrustation will occur after a period of time; with incessant heat effusion, malign sores will occur. If there is generalized heaviness, which is relieved following sweating, generalized twitching with chest pain will occur after some time. In addition, there will also be sweating above the lower back, no sweating in the lower body, slackness and pain of the lower back and hips, a sensation of something in the skin, and in severe cases, an inability to eat, generalized body pain, vexation, agitation, and inhibited urination. This is yellow sweat. *Guì Zhī Jiā Huáng Qí Tāng* rules it.

桂枝芍藥生薑（ 各三兩 ）甘草黄芪（ 各二兩 ）大棗（ 十二枚 ）

guì zhī	桂枝	9g
sháo yào	芍藥	9g
shēng jiāng	生薑	9g
gān cǎo	甘草	6g
huáng qí	黄芪	6g
dà zǎo	大棗	12 pcs

上六味，以水八升，煮取三升，溫服一升，須臾啜熱稀粥一升餘以助藥力，溫覆，取微汗；若不汗，更服 。

Simmer the six ingredients above in 1,600ml of water, until reduced to 600ml, and take 200ml warm. After a short period of time, drink a little more than 200ml of warm, thin rice gruel to en-

60. Although the characters *róng qì* 榮氣, used here, signify construction qì, the *Jīn Guì Yào Lüè* uses the characters *láo qì* 勞氣, which means taxation qì. Translators note: I have chosen to translate this as taxation qì in keeping with the original text.

hance the strength of the medicinals. Cover up to keep warm and to obtain a mild sweat. If there is no sweating, take another dose of the decoction.

Song 歌曰:

黃汗都由鬱熱來，
歷詳變態費心裁；
桂枝原劑耆加二，
啜粥重溫令鬱
久鬱變證，
從汗而達。開 。

All [cases] of yellow sweat are due to depressed heat.
Thoroughly investigate the pattern changes and carefully differentiate.
Six grams of *huáng qí* is added to the original *Guì Zhī Tāng* formula.
Sipping gruel to enhance warmth opens depression.
[It is] enduring depression [which] transforms into [this] pattern.
By [causing one to] sweat, it will be outthrust.

Commentary by [Chén] Yuánxī 男元犀按:

黃本於鬱熱，得汗不能透徹，則鬱熱不能外達。桂枝湯雖調和營衛，啜粥可令作汗，然恐其力量不及，故又加黃芪以助之，黃芪善走皮膚，故前方得苦酒之酸而能收，此方得薑、桂之辛而能發也。

The origin of yellowing is due to depressed heat. Simply inducing sweat is unable to penetrate [it], so as a result, depressed heat is unable to outthrust into the exterior. Even though *Guì Zhī Tāng* harmonizes construction and defense, drinking gruel can bring forth a sweat, and because the strength is inferior, *huáng qí* is added to reinforce it. *Huáng qí* is good at penetrating the skin. The previous formula used the sourness of vinegar to astringe, while this formula uses acrid *shēng jiāng* and *guì zhī* in order to effuse.

前方止汗，是治黃汗之正病法；此方令微汗，是治黃汗之變證法。

The previous formula stops sweating, and is the method [of choice] for treating a regular case of yellow sweating disease. This formula causes a mild sweat, and is the alternate method [of choice] for treating patterns of yellow sweating.

桂甘薑棗麻辛附子湯

Guì Gān Jiāng Zǎo Má Xīn Fù Zǐ Tāng

Cinnamon Twig, Licorice, Ginger, Date, Ephedra, Asarum, and Aconite Decoction[61]

治氣分，心下堅，大如盤，邊如旋盤，此湯主之。

A treatment for qì aspect [disease] with hardness below the heart the size of a platter with edges that resemble an overturned platter.[62] This decoction rules it.

桂枝生薑（各三兩）細辛甘草麻黃（各二兩）附子（一枚，炮）大棗（十二枚）

guì zhī	桂枝		9g
shēng jiāng	生薑		9g
xì xīn	細辛		6g
gān cǎo	甘草		6g
má huáng	麻黃		6g
fù zǐ	附子	blast-fried	1 pc
dà zǎo	大棗		12 pcs

上七味，以水七升，先煮麻黃，去上沫，內諸藥，煮取二升，分溫三服，當汗出，如蟲行皮中，即愈。

Of the seven ingredients above, first simmer the *má huáng* in 1,400ml of water and remove the foam collecting on top. Add the remaining ingredients and simmer until reduced to 400ml. Divide and take warm in three doses. [Afterwards] there should be sweating, with a sensation of insects crawling in the skin, which indicates recovery.

61. Also known as: *Guì Zhī Qù Sháo Yào Jiā Má Huáng Xì Xīn Fù Zǐ Tāng* 桂枝去芍藥加麻黃細辛附子湯 (Cinnamon Twig Decoction minus Peony plus Ephedra, Asarum, and Aconite).

62. Overturned platter: In the original text (*Jīn Guì Yào Lüè*) this is written as "an overturned cup."

Song 歌曰:

心下如盤
邊若杯，如旋杯。
辛甘麻二附全枚，
薑桂三兩棗十二，
氣分須從氣轉回 。
大氣一轉，結氣乃散。

Below the heart, [one feels] as if there [is hardness] like a platter,
with edges [resembling] a cup **like an overturned cup.**
Six grams each of *xì xīn, gān cǎo, má huáng,* and a whole piece of *fù zǐ.*
Nine grams of *gān jiāng* and *guì zhī,* and twelve pieces of *dà zǎo,*
for [disease in] the qì aspect [one] must treat the qì.
When the great qì shifts, [the] bind will immediately dissipate.

Comparison 參:

此證是心腎交病，上不能降，下不能升，日積月累，如鐵石難破。方中用麻黃、桂枝、生薑以攻其上，附子、細辛以攻其下，甘草、大棗補中焦以運其氣。㢠上下之氣交通，而病可愈，所謂大氣一轉，其結乃散也。

This pattern [belongs to] a heart and kidney interaction disease, where the upper is unable to descend, and the lower is unable to ascend. After a long period of time, it becomes hard to break like iron and stone. The formula uses *má huáng, guì zhī,* and *shēng jiāng* in order to attack the upper; *fù zǐ,* and *xì xīn* are used to attack the lower, and *gān cǎo* and *dà zǎo* to supplement the central burner in order to transport qì. Once there is interaction between the qì of the upper and lower, the disease can be cured. It is said that once the great qì shifts, [the] bind will immediately dissipate.

枳朮湯

Zhǐ Zhú Tāng

Immature Bitter Orange and Atractylodes Macrocephala Decoction

治心下堅，大如盤，邊如旋杯，水飲所作，此湯主之。

A treatment for hardness below the heart the size of a platter with edges that resemble an overturned cup. When it is due to water-rheum, this decoction rules it.

枳實（七枚）白朮（二兩）

zhǐ shí	枳實	7 pcs
bái zhú	白朮	6g

上二味，以水五升，煮取三升，分溫三服，腹中軟即當散也。

Simmer the two ingredients above in 1,000ml of water until reduced to 600ml. Divide and take warm in three doses. Once the abdomen softens, this indicates the dissipation [of water-rheum].

Song 歌曰:

心下如盤大又堅，
邪之結聚散驗其邊，
朮宜二兩枳枚七，
苦泄轉療水飲愆。

Hardness below the heart the size of a platter;
examine the edges [to check for] binding, gathering [or] dissipation of evil.
Six grams *bái zhú* is suitable, as is seven pieces of *zhǐ shí*,
for bitterness drains [in order] to shift [qì] and treats the transgression of water-rheum.

Commentary by [Chén] Wèi 蔚按:

言水飲，所以別於氣分也。氣無形，以辛甘散之；水有形，以苦洩之。方中取白朮之溫以健運，枳實之寒以消導，意深哉。

[When] discussing the differences between water-rheum and qì aspect [diseases], qì is formless, and is dissipated with acrid-sweet [substances], while water has form, which is drained with bitterness. Within the formula, the warmth of *bái zhú* is used to fortify the transportation [function], and the coldness of *zhǐ shì* is used to guide out and disperse; its meaning is deep indeed!

此方與上方互服，亦是妙法。

Giving this formula alongside the previous formula is also a wonderful method.

附方
Fù Fāng
Attached Formulas

《外臺》防己黃芪湯
Wài Tái Fáng Jǐ Huáng Qí Tāng
Fáng Jǐ and Astragalus Decoction from the *Wài Tái Mì Yào*

方見風濕。

For the formula, see [the section on] "Wind Dampness Diseases."

治風水，脈浮為在表，其人或頭汗出，表無他病，病者但下重，從腰以上為和，以下當腫及陰，難以屈伸 。

A treatment for wind-water, with a floating pulse, which indicates [that evil] is [located] in the exterior, [and although] the patient may sweat from the head, there is no exterior disease; the patient will only have heaviness in the lower body. There is no disease above the lower back, but below [the lower back] there is swelling that reaches the genitals and difficulty bending and stretching.

卷五
Volume Five

黄癉病方

Huáng Dàn Bìng Fāng

Formulas for Jaundice

茵陳蒿湯

Yīn Chén Hāo Tāng

Virgate Wormwood Decoction

歌見《傷寒》。

For the song, see the *Shāng Hán Lùn*.

治谷癉寒熱不食，食即頭眩，心胸不安，久久發黄，此湯主之。

A treatment for grain jaundice with [aversion to] cold, heat [effusion], an inability to eat, dizziness following eating, and disquietude in the heart and chest. After an extended period of time, yellowing occurs, [and] this decoction rules it.

茵陳蒿（六兩）梔子（十四枚）大黄（二兩）

yīn chén hāo	茵陳蒿	18g
zhī zǐ	梔子	14 pcs
dà huáng	大黄	6g

上三味，以水一斗，先煮茵陳，減六升，內二味，煮取三升，去滓，分溫三服。小便當利，尿如皂角汁狀，色正赤，一宿腹減，黄從小便去也。

For the three ingredients above, use 2,000ml of water. First simmer the *yīn chén hāo* until reduced to 1,200ml, add the other ingredients, and [simmer] until reduced to 600ml. Remove the dregs, divide and take warm, three doses per day. The urination should be uninhibited and resemble the color of *zào jiǎo* juice, with a full red color. Overnight the size of the abdomen will reduce, as the yellowing is eliminated through the urination.

Commentary by [Chén] Yuánxī 男元犀按:

太陰，濕土也；陽明，燥土也。經云：谷入於胃，游溢精氣，其上輸下轉，藉脾氣之能也。谷癉者，食谷入胃，脾氣不輸，濕與熱並，久則熏蒸成黃，黃成則榮衛流行之機為之阻而不利，故有寒熱不食之病。

Tàiyīn is damp earth. Yángmíng is dry earth. The classic[63] says: Grains enter the stomach, and emerge as essential qì, which are then transported upwards, and downwards by means of the spleen qì function. In grain jaundice, food and grains enter the stomach, and spleen qì is unable to transport it, so dampness and heat combine, and after some time, fume and steam [one another] becoming jaundice [yellowing]. Jaundice is formed, and as a result, the nutritive and defense-spreading mechanism is obstructed and inhibited, causing a disease of cold and heat with an inability to eat.

經云：食入於陰，長氣於陽。食即頭眩，心胸不安者，谷入於胃，挾濁氣以上乾也。主以茵陳蒿湯者，茵陳稟冬令寒水之氣，寒能勝熱；佐以梔子味苦瀉火，色黃入胃；挾大黃以滌胃腸之鬱熱，使之屈曲下行，則谷癉之邪悉從二便而解矣。

The classic[64] says: Food enters [as] yīn, and [supports the] growth of qì in the yáng. After eating there is immediately dizziness, and disquietude in the heart and chest. Grains enter the stomach, and are complicated by turbid qì [which] assaults upwards. The ruling [formula] is *Yīn Chén Hāo Tāng*. *Yīn chén* receives the cold-water qì of winter, and its coldness can overcome heat. The assistant *zhī zǐ* has a bitter flavor, and can drain fire; it has a yellow color which enters the stomach, and with *dà huáng* can flush out depressed heat in the stomach and intestines, and cause winding and downward movement, so the evil of grain jaundice can follow the [path] of the two conveniences [urination and stools] and be eliminated!

63. *Huáng Dì Nèi Jīng Sù Wèn*, Chapter 21.

64. *Huáng Dì Nèi Jīng Sù Wèn*, Chapter 46.

硝石礬石散

Xiāo Shí Fán Shí Sǎn

Niter and Alum Powder

治黃家日晡所發熱，而反惡寒，此為女勞得之；膀胱急，少腹滿，身盡黃，額上黑，足下熱，因作黑癉，其腹脹如水狀，大便必黑，時溏，此女勞之病，非水病也。腹滿者難治，此散主之。

A treatment for patients [suffering from] yellowing who typically have late afternoon heat effusion, but instead have an aversion to cold; this is sexual taxation jaundice. Urgency of the bladder, lower abdominal fullness, generalized yellowing, darkening of the forehead, [and] heat in the soles of the feet are due to black jaundice. Patients with abdominal distention that resembles a water [pattern] will have black stools which are often sloppy; this indicates sexual taxation jaundice, and is not a water disease. Those with abdominal fullness are hard to treat [and] this powder rules it.

硝石（ 熬黃 ）礬石（ 燒，等分 ）

xiāo shí	硝石	toasted until yellow	equal parts
fán shí	礬石	roasted	equal parts

上二味為散，大麥粥汁和，服方寸匕，日三服。病隨大小便去，小便正黃，大便正黑，是其候也。

Process the two ingredients above into a powder, and take one gram, combined with barley gruel, three doses per day. The disease will be eliminated through the bowel movements and urination, in the form of yellow urine and black stools.

Song 歌曰:

身黃額黑
漸及一身之黃俱黑
足如烘，腹脹如水狀，
便溏便溏而色黑晡熱叢，
日晡熱，以申屬膀胱，

酉屬腎也。
等分礬硝和麥汁，
女勞癉病奪天工。

Generalized yellowing with darkness of the forehead,
yellowing with darkness gradually reaching the whole body,
feet [which feel] as if baked, abdominal distention, **resembling a water pattern,**
sloppy stools, **sloppy stools [that are] black in color,** and late afternoon heat.
With late afternoon heat, the period of *shēn*[65] belongs to the bladder,
and the period of *yǒu*[66] belongs to the kidneys.
Equal parts *fán shí* and *xiāo shí* with barley juice,
and sexual taxation jaundice disease is plundered [by the] heavenly practitioner.

Quotation by Xú Zhōngkě 徐忠可云:

硝能散虛鬱之熱，為體輕脫，而寒不傷脾；礬能卻水，而所到之處邪不復侵，如紙既礬，即不受水滲也。以大麥粥調服，益土以勝水，合而用之，則散鬱熱，解腎毒。其與氣血陰陽汗下補瀉等法，毫不相涉，所以為佳。

Xiāo shí can dissipate vacuous depressed heat, causing [it to be] lightly shed from the body, while its coldness will not damage the spleen. *Fán shí* is able to eliminate water, so [water] evil is not able to invade wherever [*fán shí*] goes, and like paper, *fán shí* does not allow for seepage of water. These [medicinals] are taken mixed with barley gruel, which boosts earth in order to overcome water, and when all are combined, can dissipate depressed heat, and resolve kidney toxicity. Here, there are no methods that involve qì, blood, yīn, yáng, sweating, precipitating, supplementing or draining in the least. However, it is [still] an excellent [formula].

65. From 3-5pm.
66. From 5-7pm.

梔子大黃湯

Zhī Zǐ Dà Huáng Tāng

Gardenia and Rhubarb Decoction

治酒癉，心中懊憹，或熱痛者，此湯主之。

A treatment for liquor jaundice, with anguish in the heart, or heat pain; this decoction rules it.

梔子（十四枚）大黃（二兩）枳實（五枚）豉（一升）

zhī zǐ	梔子	14 pcs
dà huáng	大黃	6g
zhǐ shí	枳實	5 pcs
chǐ	豉	200ml

上四味，以水六升，煮取二升，分溫三服。

Simmer the four ingredients above in 1,200ml of water until reduced to 400ml. Divide and take warm, three doses per day.

Song 歌曰:

酒癉懊憹鬱熱蒸，
大黃二兩豉盈升，
梔子十四枳枚五，
上下分消要順承。

Liquor jaundice [with] anguish and steaming of depressed heat;
dà huáng six grams, and *dàn dòu chǐ* at 200ml;
fourteen pieces of *zhī zǐ* and five of *zhǐ shí*.
Above and below are separately dispersed and there is smooth coordination [downwards].

Commentary by [Chén] Yuánxī 元犀按:

梔子、豆豉徹熱於上，枳實、大黃除實去滿於下，此所謂上下分消，順承熱氣也。

Zhī zǐ, and *dòu chǐ* penetrate heat in the upper, while *zhǐ shí* and *dà huáng* eliminate repletion and remove fullness in the lower. This is what is meant by separately dispersing the upper and lower, and smoothly coordinating heat qì [downwards].

Quotation by Xú Zhōngkě 徐忠可云:

因酒徒陰分大傷，故不用燥藥以耗其津，亦不用滲藥以竭其液，謂熱散則濕不能留也。凡治濕熱而兼燥者，於此可悟。

Because liquor greatly damages the yīn aspect to no avail, dry medicinals are therefore not used [to avoid] consuming liquids. In addition, percolating medicinals are also not used [to avoid] exhausting fluids. It is said that [once] heat is dissipated, dampness would be unable to be retained. One should comprehend that [this method applies to] all treatments of dampness and heat with concurrent dryness.

桂枝加黃芪湯

Guì Zhī Jiā Huáng Qí Tāng

Cinnamon Twig Decoction plus Astragalus

歌見水氣病中。

For the song, see [the section on] "Water Qì Diseases."

治黃癉病，但當利其小便。假令脈浮者，當以汗解之，宜此湯。

When treating jaundice, [one] simply needs to disinhibit urination. If the pulse is floating, sweating should be promoted to resolve [the condition], and this decoction is appropriate.

桂枝（三兩）芍藥（三兩）甘草（二兩）生薑（三兩）大棗（十二枚）黃芪（二兩）

guì zhī	桂枝	9g
sháo yào	芍藥	9g
gān cǎo	甘草	6g
shēng jiāng	生薑	9g
dà zǎo	大棗	12 pcs
huáng qí	黃芪	6g

上六味，以水八升，煮取三升，溫服一升，須臾飲熱稀粥一升餘，以助藥力，溫服取微汗；若不汗，更服。

Simmer the six ingredients above in 1,600ml of water until reduced to 600ml, and take 200ml warm. After some time, take a little more than 200ml of warm, thin rice gruel to enhance the strength of the medicinals. Cover up to keep warm and to obtain a mild sweat. If there is no sweating, take another dose of the decoction.

Commentary by [Chén] Yuánxī 男元犀按:

黄瘅症多由濕熱內鬱而成，為病在內也。鬱在內者，宜內解，故曰當利其小便，小便通則所鬱皆去矣。假令脈浮者，病在肌表也，當外解，故曰當以汗解之。桂枝湯解肌發表，加黄芪助之，以黄芪有發汗退黄之專長也。

Jaundice patterns are typically caused by the internal depression of dampness and heat, so [therefore] this is an internal disease. [With] depression in the interior, it is appropriate to resolve the interior; therefore it is said that [one] should disinhibit urination. Once the urine is free, all which is depressed will be eliminated. For example, [when the] pulse is floating, the disease is in the fleshy exterior, and the exterior should be resolved, hence the saying that [one] must use sweating [to] resolve [the exterior]. *Guì Zhī Tāng* resolves the fleshy exterior, and the addition of *huáng qí* assists it [in this function], as *huáng qí* has the specific function of promoting sweat in order to abate jaundice.

豬膏發煎

Zhū Gāo Fā Jiān

Pork Lard and Human Hair Brew

治諸黃癉病 。

A treatment for all jaundice diseases.

豬膏（ 半斤 ）亂發（ 如雞子大三枚 ）

zhū gāo	豬膏		24g
luàn fà	亂發	the size of a large chicken egg	3 pcs

上二味，和膏中煎之，發消藥成，分再服，病從小便出 。

Mix the two ingredients above, and boil until the hair is completely dissolved. Divide and take in two doses. The condition will be relieved through urination.

《千金》云：太醫校尉史脫家婢黃病服此，胃中燥糞下便差，神驗。

The *Qiān Jīn Fāng* retells [a case] of Shǐ Tuō, an imperial physician who administered this formula to his personal maidservant who had contracted jaundice. Dry stools were present in the stomach, and [following] precipitation [the condition] was relieved, and the effect was divine!

Song 歌曰：

諸黃腹鼓大便堅，
古有豬膏八兩傳，
亂發三枚雞子大，
發消藥熟始停煎 。

[In] all [cases] of yellowing with abdominal drum [distention] and hard stools,
the ancients' knowledge of using twenty-four grams of *zhū gāo* has been handed down.

Three pieces of *luàn fà* the size of a chicken egg,
boiled until all the hair is dissolved.

Commentary by [Chén] Yuánxī 男元犀按:

豬膏主潤燥，發灰主通小便，故《神農本草經》有自還神化句最妙，謂發為血餘，乃水精奉心化血所生。今取以煉服，仍能入至陰之臟，助水精以上奉心臟之神，以化其血也。沈自南謂寒濕入於血分，久而生熱，鬱蒸氣血不利，證顯津枯血燥，皮膚黃而暗晦，即爲陰黃，當以此治之。且熱鬱既久陰血無有不傷，治者皆宜兼滋其陰，故曰諸黃主之。

Zhū gāo rules the moistening of dryness, and *luàn fà* rules the freeing of urination. In the *Shén Nóng Běn Cǎo Jīng* there is a very ingenious and exemplary sentence, which states that hair is the surplus of blood, [whereby] water essence is received by the heart and transformed into blood. Nowadays [this formula] is taken processed, [but is] still capable of entering the yīn organs. Thereby water essence is assisted in its ascent in order to be received by the spirit of the heart and be transformed into blood. Chén Zìnán[67] says that when cold and dampness enter the blood aspect, after some time they will generate heat, which will depress and steam the qì and blood leaving them inhibited, resulting in a pattern of desiccation of liquid and blood dryness. The skin will turn yellow and dark, which is referred to as yīn yellowing, and [one] should [utilize] this treatment [method]. Moreover, [with] enduring depressed heat, which has damaged yīn and blood, it is therefore appropriate to simultaneously enrich the yīn, which is why it is said that [this formula] rules the treatment of all jaundice [diseases].

Additional Commentary 又按:

又按：時醫惑於以人補人之說，每遇虛證，輒以紫河車配藥。余幼時隨待，聞家君與客常談及紫河車一物。

Others have said that whenever a vacuous pattern is encountered [one should] always combine [the medicinals] with *zǐ hé chē*. In my childhood, I frequently heard the mentioning of *zǐ hé chē* in discussions between my father and his visitors.

67. Chén Zìnán 沈自南, a *Qīng* Dynasty physician.

曰：某也服此，今反肌肉羸瘦，某也服此，病反增劇。吾行道數十年，見有用紫河車者，未嘗一效。余默識之。今省中行道輩，遇病人家有餘貲或病證虛弱火熾等證，即曰：非紫河車不能成功也。嗚呼！是醫也而能活人乎？是藥也而能活人乎？

My father said that [when] some take this [medicinal], their flesh [becomes] severely emaciated, [while] others [when taking this medicinal] on the contrary, their disease exacerbates. In over tens of years of [my own] medical practice, I have yet to see the effect of *zǐ hé chē*. For [this is] my own silent recollection. Presently, local contemporaries when encountering [patients] who are wealthy or [ones] with signs of vacuity weakness or intense fire, would say, that *zǐ hé chē* simply must be used [for this formula] to be effective. Alas! Can these physicians save lives? Can this medicinal save lives?

茵陳五苓散

Yīn Chén Wǔ Líng Sǎn

Five-Substance Powder with Poria plus Capillaris Decoction

治黄癉病。

A treatment for jaundice disease.

茵陳（ 十分 ）五苓散（ 五分 ）

yīn chén	茵陳	10 parts
wǔ líng sǎn	五苓散	5 parts

上二味和，先食飲服方寸匕，日三服。

Combine the two ingredients above, and take one gram before meals, three doses per day.

Song 歌曰:

癉病傳來兩解方，
表裏兩解。
茵陳末入五苓嘗，
五苓五分專行水，
茵陳十分卻退黄。

[When] jaundice arrives, [use] a formula for double resolution.
Resolving both the exterior and interior.
Powdered *yīn chén* added to *Wǔ Líng Sǎn*.
Five parts *Wǔ Líng Sǎn* specifically moves water
[while] ten parts *yīn chén* eliminates and abates jaundice.

Commentary by [Chén] Yuánxī 男元犀按：

五苓散功專發汗利水，助脾轉輸；茵陳蒿功專治濕退黃，合五苓散為解鬱利濕之用也。蓋黃癉病由濕熱瘀鬱，熏蒸成黃，非茵陳蒿推陳致新，不足以除熱退黃；非五苓散轉輸利濕，不足以發汗行水。二者之用，取其表裏兩解，爲治黃之良劑也。

The function of *Wǔ Líng Sǎn* is specifically to promote sweating, disinhibit urination, and assist in the spleen's activity of transportation. *Yīn chén hāo* is specifically used to treat dampness and abate jaundice, and [when] combined with *Wǔ Líng Sǎn,* they are used to resolve depression and disinhibit dampness. Jaundice is due to dampness and heat stasis and depression steaming [upwards] thus causing yellowing. Unless *yīn chén hāo* is used to push out the old to make room for the new, [one] cannot eliminate heat and abate jaundice. [In addition] unless *Wǔ Líng Sǎn* is used to shift and transport water, [one] cannot promote sweating and move water. By using these two together, both the interior and exterior are resolved, making this an excellent formula to treat jaundice.

大黄硝石湯

Dà Huáng Xiāo Shí Tāng

Rhubarb and Niter Decoction

治黄癉腹滿，小便不利而赤，自汗出，此為表和裏實，當下之，宜此湯。

A treatment for jaundice with abdominal fullness, inhibited red urination, and spontaneous sweating, which indicates a harmonized exterior and interior repletion. Precipitation should be used, and this decoction is suitable.

大黄黄柏硝石（各四兩）梔子（十五枚）

dà huáng	大黄	12g
huáng bǎi	黄柏	12g
xiāo shí	硝石	12g
zhī zǐ	梔子	15 pcs

上四味，以水六升，煮取二升，去滓，內硝更煮取一升，頓服。

Simmer the four ingredients above in 1,200ml of water until reduced to 400ml. Remove the dregs, add the *xiāo shí*, and simmer until reduced to 200ml. Take as one single dose.

Song 歌曰:

自汗表無邪也
屎難大便難腹滿時，
表和裏實貴隨宜；
硝黄四兩柏同數，
十五枚梔任指麾。

When [there is] spontaneous sweating, **absence of evil in the exterior**
and difficult stools **difficult bowel movements,** with abdominal fullness,
the exterior is harmonious and the interior is replete, nobly comply [with a] suitable [treatment].

Twelve grams of *xiāo shí* and *dà huáng*, the same of *huáng bǎi*,
while fifteen pieces of *zhī zǐ* are commanded.

Commentary by [Chén] Yuánxī 男元犀按：

黄癉病濕熱交鬱，不得外通，今自汗出者，外已通也。腹滿小便不利而赤者，濕熱仍實於裏也。實者當下，故用大黄除滿去實，硝石領熱氣下趨二便，又以黄柏除滿退黄，梔子散熱解鬱。濕熱散，二便調，則裏氣亦和矣。

Jaundice disease [is due to] the merging and depression of damp and heat, which are unable to flow freely to the outside. Now there is spontaneous sweating, [which signifies] that the exterior is already free. Abdominal fullness with red, inhibited urination [means that] dampness and heat are still replete in the interior. This repletion should be precipitated, therefore *dà huáng* is used to eliminate fullness and repletion. *Xiāo shí* leads heat qì downwards through the stools and urine. *Huáng bǎi* is also used to eliminate fullness and abate jaundice. *Zhī zǐ* dissipates heat and resolves depression. When dampness and heat are dissipated, and the stools and urine are regulated, then interior qì will also be harmonized.

小半夏湯
Xiǎo Bàn Xià Tāng
Minor Pinellia Decoction

歌見痰飲。

For the song, see [the section on] "Phlegm-rheum Diseases."

治黃癉病，小便色不變，欲自利，腹滿而喘，不可除熱，熱除必噦。噦者，此湯主之。

A treatment for jaundice disease where the color of the urine is unchanged and there is a tendency towards spontaneous diarrhea, with abdominal fullness and panting. [One cannot] eliminate heat as this will result in retching. For retching, this decoction rules it.

半夏（一升）生薑（半斤）

bàn xià	半夏	200ml
shēng jiāng	生薑	24g

上二味，以水七升，煮取一升半，分溫再服。

Simmer the two ingredients above in 1,400ml of water until reduced to 300ml. Divide and take warm in two doses.

Commentary by [Chén] Yuánxī 元犀按:

《傷寒論》云：瘀熱在裏，身必發黃。此云小便色不變，欲自利者，可知內無瘀熱矣。蓋喘滿屬中氣虛弱，故曰不可除熱。師恐後人誤投寒劑傷中，故立小半夏湯以救誤治也。用半夏和胃以鎮逆，生薑溫理中臟，中溫則升降自如，而喘滿嘔逆自愈。

The *Shāng Hán Lùn* says: [When there is] static heat in the interior, there must be yellowing of the body. Here it says that the color of the urine should not change, and [if there is] a desire to naturally disinhibit, we know that there is no static heat in the interior. In all [cases] of panting and fullness [due to] central qì vacuity, it is said that we cannot eliminate heat. The master, fearing that later generations would falsely use cold formulas and damage the center, therefore established [*Xiǎo*] *Bàn Xià Tāng* in order to rescue from erroneous treatments. *Bàn xià* is used to harmonize the stomach in order to settle counterflow. *Shēng jiāng* warms the interior central viscera. [Once] the center is warm, upbearing and downbearing will [move] freely, and panting, fullness, retching, and counterflow are cured on their own.

Additional Commentary 又按:

若中虛發黄者，余每用理中湯、真武湯等加茵陳蒿，多效。

If jaundice is due to central vacuity, I always achieve great results using *Lǐ Zhōng Tāng* or *Zhēn Wǔ Tāng* with the addition of *yīn chén hāo.*

小柴胡湯

Xiǎo Chái Hú Tāng

Minor Bupleurum Decoction

歌見《傷寒》。

For the song, see the *Shāng Hán Lùn.*

治諸黃腹痛而嘔者，宜此湯主之。

A treatment for all jaundice [diseases] with abdominal pain and retching, this decoction is appropriate and rules it.

柴胡（半斤）黃芩（三兩）人參（三兩）甘草（三兩）半夏（半斤）生薑（三兩）大棗（十二枚）

chái hú	柴胡	24g
huáng qín	黃芩	9g
rén shēn	人參	9g
gān cǎo	甘草	9g
bàn xià	半夏	24g
shēng jiāng	生薑	9g
dà zǎo	大棗	12 pcs

上七味，以水一斗二升，煮取六升，去滓，再煎取三升，溫服一升，日三服。

Simmer the seven ingredients above in 2,400ml of water until reduced to 1,200ml. Remove the dregs and boil again until reduced to 600ml. Take 200ml warm, three doses per day.

Commentary by [Chén] Yuánxī 男元犀按:

嘔者，胃氣不和也。腹痛者，木邪犯胃也。小柴胡湯達木鬱，和胃氣，使中樞運則嘔痛止而黃退矣。非小柴胡湯可概治諸黃也。

Retching [is the result of] the disharmony of the stomach qì. Abdominal pain is [the result of] wood evil invading the stomach. *Xiǎo Chái Hú Tāng* outthrusts depressed wood, harmonizes the stomach, and causes movement of the central pivot, which will stop the retching and pain, and abate jaundice. [However], it is not the case that *Xiǎo Chái Hú Tāng* is capable of treating all [cases] of jaundice.

小建中湯
Xiǎo Jiàn Zhōng Tāng
Minor Center-Strengthening Decoction

歌見《傷寒》。

For the song, see the *Shāng Hán Lùn.*

治男子黃，小便自利，當與虛勞小建中湯。

A treatment for males with jaundice and spontaneous urination, *Xiǎo Jiàn Zhōng Tāng* for deficiency taxation should be given.

桂枝（三兩，去皮）甘草（三兩，炙）大棗（十二枚）芍藥（六兩）生薑（三兩）膠飴（一升）

guì zhī	桂枝	bark removed	9g
gān cǎo	甘草	honey-fried	9g
dà zǎo	大棗		12 pcs
sháo yào	芍藥		18g
shēng jiāng	生薑		9g
jiāo yí	膠飴		200ml

上六味，以水七升，煮取三升，去滓，內膠飴，更上微火消解，溫服一升，日三服。嘔家不可用建中湯，以甜故也。

Simmer the six ingredients above in 1,400ml of water until reduced to 600ml. Remove the dregs, add the *jiāo yí,* and again place on low heat until [the *jiāo yí*] is dispersed. Take 200ml warm, three doses per day. **Retching patients cannot take *Jiàn Zhōng Tāng* because it is too sweet.**

Commentary by [Chén] Wèi 男蔚按:

此言土虛而現出黄色也。虛極者，宜補土之母，四逆輩可與間服。然單言男子，謂婦人血瘀發黄，尚有桃仁承氣湯法也。苟屬虛黄，亦宜以此湯加當歸、益母葉之類也。

Here [the text] is describing the emergence of jaundice [due to] vacuity of the earth. In extreme vacuity, it is appropriate to supplement the mother of earth, and the *Sì Nì* family [of formulas] can be given alongside [this formula]. However, [the text] simply mentions males, [so for] woman with jaundice due to blood stasis, the method would be [to administer] *Táo Rén Chéng Qì Tāng*. If it were a case of vacuity jaundice, then this decoction would be appropriate with the addition of medicinals such as *dāng guī* and *yì mǔ cǎo*.

附方
Fù Fāng
Attached Formulas

瓜蒂散
Guā Dì Sǎn
Melon Stalk Decoction

歌見《傷寒》。

For the song, see the *Shāng Hán Lùn.*

治諸黃。

Treats various [kinds of] jaundice [diseases].

瓜蒂（一分，熬黃）赤小豆（一分，煮）

guā dì	瓜蒂	boiled until yellow	1 part
chì xiǎo dòu	赤小豆	cooked	1 part

上二味，杵為散，以香豉七合煮取汁，和散一錢匕，溫服之，不吐者少加之，以快吐乃度而止。亡血及虛者，不可與之。

Process the two ingredients above by pestling them into a powder, and take one *qián*-spoon full with a warm decoction made from 140ml of *xiāng dòu.* If the [patient] does not vomit, increase the dosage and stop once they are vomiting. This [formula] cannot be given to [patients] with blood collapse or vacuity.

Commentary by [Chén] Yuánxī 男元犀按：

瓜蒂散《傷寒論》三見，俱主胸中之病。《金匱》取之附治諸黃，何也？蓋黃乃濕熱相並，鬱蒸不得外越，用瓜蒂散吐而越之，使上膈開而下竅達，濕熱之邪自有出路矣，故曰治諸黃。

Guā Dì Sǎn is mentioned three times in the *Shāng Hán Lùn,* mainly for diseases in the chest. Why is it an additional [formula] for the treatment of all [kinds of] jaundice in the *Jīn Guì* [*Yào Lüè*]? All jaundice [is the result of the] depression and steaming of dampness and heat, which mix together and are unable to thrust out externally. Use *Guā Dì Sǎn* to [cause] vomiting [which] thrusts out [evils]. It causes opening [both] above the diaphragm and in the lower orifices, creating a path from which dampness and heat evils may be expelled. This is the reason it treats all jaundice.

《千金》麻黃醇酒湯
Qiān Jīn Má Huáng Chún Jiǔ Tāng
Ephedra and Wine Decoction from the *Qiān Jīn Yào Fāng*

治黃癉。

A treatment for jaundice.

麻黃（三兩）

má huáng　麻黃　9g

上一味，以美酒五升，煮取二升半，頓服盡。冬月用酒，春日用水煮之。

Add *má huáng* to 1,000ml of clear liquor, and simmer until reduced to 500ml. Take as one single dose. In the winter simmer with liquor, and in the spring use water.

Song 歌曰:

黃癉病由鬱熱成，
驅邪解表仗雄兵；
五升酒煮麻三兩，
春換水兮去酒烹。

Jaundice is the result of depressed heat;
expelling evils and resolving the exterior [is likened] to the reliance on a powerful army;
simmer nine grams *má huáng* with 1,000ml of liquor,
[and in] the spring use water instead of liquor.

Commentary by [Chén] Yuánxī 男元犀按:

麻黃輕清走表，乃氣分之藥，主無汗表實症。黃癉病不離濕熱之邪，用麻黃醇酒湯者，以黃在肌表榮衛之間，非麻黃不能走肌表，非美酒不能通榮衛，故用酒煮以助麻黃發汗，汗出則榮衛通，有內蘊之邪悉從外解耳。

Má huáng is light and clear and penetrates the exterior. It is a qì aspect medicinal, which rules exterior repletion patterns with absence of sweating. Jaundice is considered to be linked to dampness and heat evils. Use *Má Huáng Chún Jiǔ Tāng* in order [to treat] jaundice located in between the fleshy exterior and the nutritive and defense. Without *má huáng*, [one] would be unable to move the fleshy exterior, and unless clear liquor is used, [one] would be unable to free the nutritive and defense. Therefore, *má huáng* is boiled in clear liquor in order to assist in [its function] of promoting sweat, as when sweat flows, then the nutritive and defense will be free, and we would know that the evil which is hidden internally will resolve through the exterior.

驚悸吐衄下血方

Jīng Jì Tǔ Nǜ Xià Xiě Fāng

Formulas for Fright Palpitations, Blood Ejection, Nosebleeds, and Descent of Blood

桂枝去芍藥加蜀漆牡蠣龍骨救逆湯

Guì Zhī Qù Sháo Yào Jiā Shǔ Qī Mǔ Lì Long Gǔ Jiù Nì Tāng

Cinnamon Twig Counterflow Stemming Decoction
minus Peony plus Dichroa Leaf, Oyster Shell, and Dragon Bone.

歌見《傷寒》。

For the song, see the *Shāng Hán Lùn.*

治火邪者，此湯主之。

A treatment for fire evil, this decoction rules it.

桂枝（三兩，去皮）甘草（二兩，炙）生薑（三兩，切）牡蠣（五兩，熬）龍骨（四兩）大棗（十二枚）蜀漆（三兩，洗去腥）

guì zhī	桂枝	bark removed	9g
gān cǎo	甘草	honey-fried	6g
shēng jiāng	生薑	cut	9g
mǔ lì	牡蠣	boiled [in salt water and then toasted]	15g
lóng gǔ	龍骨		12g
dà zǎo	大棗		12 pcs
shǔ qī	蜀漆	wash to remove the fishy [smell]	9g

上為末，以水一斗二升，先煮蜀漆，減二升，內諸藥，煮取三升，去滓，溫服一升。

Pound [all seven ingredients] into a powder. First simmer the *shǔ qī* in 2,400ml of water until reduced by 400ml. Add the other ingredients and simmer until reduced to 600ml. Remove the dregs and take 200ml warm.

Commentary by [Chén] Xīndiǎn 孫男心典稟按：

舉火邪冠於方首，示人治血先治火也，又恐治火專主寒滯之品，故拈出此方不寒不滯以立榜樣，意深哉！《傷寒論》注解甚詳，不必再釋。

Fire evil is the first [thing mentioned] before the formula. People are instructed [that] in order to treat the blood, fire must be treated first, but out of fear [they] use cold, stagnating ingredients to treat the fire. Therefore [Zhāng Zhòngjǐng] grasped this formula, which is neither cold nor stagnating to treat [this pattern]. Its meaning is deep indeed! The explanation in the *Shāng Hán Lùn* is quite detailed, so there is no need for further explanation.

半夏麻黃丸
Bàn Xià Má Huáng Wán
Pinellia and Ephedra Pill

治心下悸者，此丸主之。

A treatment for palpitations below the heart; this pill rules it.

半夏麻黃（各等分）

bàn xià	半夏	equal parts
má huáng	麻黃	equal parts

上二味末之，煉蜜為丸小豆大，飲服三丸，日三服。

Process equal parts of the two ingredients above into a powder and combine with refined honey to form pills the size of small beans. Take three pills, three times daily.

Song 歌曰:

心下悸都緣飲氣維，
夏麻等分蜜丸醫；
一升一降存其意，
神化原來不可知。

All palpitations **below** the heart are the result of rheum qì.
Equal parts *bàn xià* and *má huáng* made into honey pill medicine.
The significance [of the formula is that] one upbears and the other downbears.
[One] would not [have] known how divine it would turn out.

Quotation by Yóu Zàijīng 尤在涇云:

半夏蠲飲氣，麻黃發陽氣，妙在作丸與服，緩以圖之。則麻黃之辛甘，不能發越津氣，而但能升陽氣；即半夏之苦辛，亦不特蠲除飲氣，而並和養中氣。非仲景神明善變者，其孰能與於此哉？

Bàn xià eliminates rheum qì, and *má huáng* effuses yáng qì. The ingenuity lies in the processing and administration of the pills, which [function] to moderately resolve [the condition]. The acrid and sweet [flavor] of *má huáng* is unable to diffuse liquid qì, and can only upbear yáng qì. In addition, the bitter and acrid [flavor] of *bàn xià* not only eliminates rheum qì, but also harmonizes and nourishes center qì. Who could ever conceive such [a formula, besides the] bright and adaptable Zhòngjǐng?

柏葉湯
Bǎi Yè Tāng
Arborvitae Leaf Decoction

治吐血不止者，此湯主之。

A treatment for incessant vomiting of blood; this decoction rules it.

柏葉乾薑（各三兩）艾（三把）

bǎi yè	柏葉	9g
gān jiāng	乾薑	9g
ài	艾	3 handfuls

上三味，以水五升，取馬通汁一升合煮，取一升，分溫再服。

Simmer the three ingredients above in 1,000ml of water and 200ml of horse manure liquid until reduced to 200ml. Divide and take warm in two doses.

《千金》加阿膠三兩，亦佳。

The *Qiān Jīn Yào Fāng* adds nine grams of *ē jiāo,* which is also excellent.

Song 歌曰:

吐血頻頻不肯休，
久吐不止,
凡一切寒溫補瀉之藥,
服之殆盡矣。
馬通升許溯源流，
熱氣伏藏於陰分,
逼血妄行不止。
馬屬火,

取其通之同氣以導之。
乾薑三兩艾三把，
二味溫散，
宣發其熱使行陽分，
則陰分之血無所逼而守其經矣。
柏葉行陰三兩求。
柏葉抑之使降，
合馬通導之使下，
則餘燼之瘀，一概蠲矣。

Repeated vomiting of blood, unwillingness to rest,
incessant chronic vomiting,
[even after] cold, warm, supplementing and draining medicinals
have been administered to no end.
200ml of horse manure liquid turns back to the source.
Hot qì is hiding and is stored in the yīn aspect,
driving incessant frenetic blood movement.
The horse is associated with fire,
and taking manure frees its similarly [natured] qì[68] and guides it [downwards].
Nine grams of *gān jiāng* and three handfuls of *ài yè*.
[These] two medicinals are warm and dissipating,
which can diffuse heat and cause it to move into the yáng aspect
then the blood of the yīn aspect is without force, [so blood] remains in the channels.
Bāi yè moves yīn, and needs to be at nine grams.
***Bāi yè* restrains and causes descent,**
and when combined with horse manure liquid, [*bāi yè* is able to] guide downwards,
so that all the static remnants can be completely eliminated.

前方歌括之小注頗詳，毋庸再釋。但愚每用前方，病家皆驚疑不能聽。今擬加減法，用生側柏五錢，乾薑（炮透）一錢五分，生艾葉三錢，水一杯半，馬通一杯，煎八分服。如無馬通，以童便代之。
馬糞用水化開，以布濾汁澄清，爲馬通水。

The small annotation in this formulas song is quite comprehensive, so there is no need for further explanation. However, every time I use this formula, patients are always full of fear and doubt, and

68. Fire.

fail to comply. These days, I have devised a modification [of the formula] using fifteen grams[69] of fresh *cè bǎi*, four and a half grams of blast-fried *gān jiāng*, and nine grams of fresh *ài yè*, boiled in one and a half cups of water with one cup of horse manure liquid, reduced to eight tenths [of a cup] and [this is then quaffed]. If horse manure liquid is not available, I substitute child's urine. Horse feces [should be] dissolved in water, and strained through a cloth leaving only the clarified liquid. This becomes horse manure liquid.

69. There is much debate regarding dosage equivalents from the *Hàn* Dynasty to present times. However, there is general consensus that following the *Táng* Dynasty (starting in 618 A.D.) the measurement of dosage changed. From this point forward, the *qián* was considered to be 3.73 grams. This commentary was written in the *Qīng* Dynasty, but the *qián* was not used in the late *Hàn* when the original text was written. Therefore I have converted and rounded down the measurement of each *qián* into three grams.

黃土湯
Huáng Tǔ Tāng
Yellow Earth Decoction

治下血，先便後血，此遠血也，亦主吐衄。

A treatment for blood precipitation, where bleeding follows the stools. This is [called] distal bleeding. [It] also rules [the treatment of] blood ejection and nosebleeds.

甘草乾地黃白朮附子（炮）阿膠黃芩（各三兩）竈中黃土（半斤）

gān cǎo	甘草		9g
gān dì huáng	乾地黃		9g
bái zhú	白朮		9g
fù zǐ	附子	blast-fried	9g
ē jiāo	阿膠		9g
huáng qín	黃芩		9g
zào zhōng huáng tǔ	竈中黃土		24g

上七味，水八升，煮取三升，分溫二服。

Simmer the seven ingredients above in 1,600ml of water until reduced to 600ml. Divide and take warm, two doses per day.

Song 歌曰：

遠血先便血續來，
半斤黃土莫徘徊；
朮膠附地芩甘草，
三兩同行血證該。
不僅治下血，而吐血、
衄血與婦人血崩等證俱該在內。

[When there is] distal bleeding [where] first there are stools followed by bleeding,
do not hesitate [to use] twenty-four grams *huáng tǔ*;

[as] together with nine grams each of *bái zhú, ē jiāo, fù zǐ, dì huáng, huáng qín,* and *gān cǎo,* [this treats] the above-mentioned blood pattern.

[This formula] not only treats blood descent, but also interior patterns of blood ejection, nosebleeds, and flooding in woman.

Quotation by Wáng Jìnsān[70] 王晉三云:

《金匱》以下血，先血後便為近血，明指脾絡受傷，日滲腸間，瘀積於下，故大便未行而血先下，主之以赤小豆利水散瘀，當歸和脾止血。若先便後血爲遠血，明指肝經別絡之血，因脾虛陽陷生濕，血亦就濕而下行，主之以竈心黄土，溫燥而去寒濕，佐以生地、阿膠、黄芩入肝以治血熱，白朮、甘草、附子扶陽補脾以治本虛。近血內瘀，專力清利；遠血因虛，故兼溫補。治出天淵，須明辨之。

The *Jīn Guì Yào Lüè* mentions blood descent, [where] there is first bleeding followed by stools, which is called proximal bleeding. This clearly indicates that the spleen network vessels have been damaged. When there is permeation [of blood] in the intestines, and stasis accumulation in the lower, the stools fail to move and blood descends first. The ruling [medicinal] *chì xiǎo dòu* disinhibits water and disperses stasis, while *dāng guī* harmonizes the spleen to stop bleeding. If there are stools first followed by bleeding, this is called distal bleeding, [which is] clearly referring to the blood of the liver channel and diverging network vessel. When the spleen is vacuous, yáng sinks and generates dampness. [Then] blood descends, following dampness. The ruling [medicinal] is *zào xīn huáng tǔ,* which is warming and drying and eliminates cold and dampness. The assistants *shēng dì huáng, ē jiāo,* and *huáng qín* enter the liver and treat blood heat. *Bái zhú, gān cǎo,* and *fù zǐ* support the yáng and supplement the spleen in order to treat the vacuous root. Proximal bleeding [is due to] interior stasis, [and] the focus must be on clearing and disinhibiting; distal bleeding is caused by vacuity, therefore [one must] simultaneously warm and supplement. [These] treatments are poles apart, so [one] must clearly differentiate them.

Commentary 按:

此方以竈心黄土易赤石脂一斤，附子易炮乾薑二兩，炮紫更妙；或加側柏葉四兩；絡熱，加鮮竹茹半斤。

In this formula, forty-eight grams of *chì shí zhī* can be used [instead of] *zào zhōng huáng tǔ.* Six grams of *páo gān jiāng* can be substituted for *fù zǐ,* [but] *páo [fù] zǐ* is even better, and twelve grams of *cè bǎi yè* can also be added. [If there is] heat in the collaterals, add twenty-four grams of fresh *zhú rú.*

70. An honored government official and physician who lived from 1698–1761.

赤小豆散

Chì Xiǎo Dòu Sǎn[71]

Rice Bean [and Chinese Angelica] Powder

歌見狐惑。

For the song, see [the section on] "Fox-creeper Diseases."

治下血先血後便，此近血也，此主之 。

A treatment for defecation with blood, where there is first bleeding followed by stools. This is called proximal bleeding [and] this [formula] rules it.

赤小豆（ 三升，浸，令芽出，曝乾 ）當歸

chì xiǎo dòu	赤小豆	soak until it sprouts, and then sun-dry.	600ml
dāng guī	當歸		no quantity given

上二味，杵為散，漿水服方寸匕，日三服 。

Process the two ingredients above by pestling them into a powder. Take one gram in fermented grain-water, three doses per day.

Commentary by [Chén] Yuánxī 男元犀按:

肝為血海，氣通胞中，主宣布之權，虛則失其權矣。曰先血後便者，肝失其統，不能下宣，致胞中之血滲入肛門也。近血者，胃接二腸，胞與腸前後，此之最近也。若胃腸受濕熱。致傷其氣，必通於胞中而迫血者也。赤小豆入心，清熱解臟毒；當歸入肝，補虛散鬱，能宣其血入於經隧也。

71. In the *Jīn Guì Yào Lüè*, *Chì Xiǎo Dòu Sǎn* is referred to as *Chì Xiǎo Dòu Dāng Guī Sǎn*.

The liver is the sea of blood and promotes the flow of qì through the womb. It rules the power of diffusion and spreading out, and in vacuity, this power is lost. [Here] it says that first there is bleeding followed by stools. This is [a result of] the liver losing control, with an inability to diffuse downwards, causing the blood in the womb to seep into the anus. [As for] proximal bleeding, the stomach is connected to the intestines, and the womb and intestines are positioned in front and behind one another, and these are the closest to each other. If the stomach and intestines contract dampness and heat, these will damage the qì, and inevitably [create] movement in the womb, which will distress the blood. ***Chì xiǎo dòu*** enters the heart, clears heat, and resolves visceral toxicity; ***dāng guī*** enters the liver, supplements vacuity, dissipates depression, and is able to diffuse the blood [and return it to] the channel passages.

瀉心湯

Xiè Xīn Tāng

Heart-Draining Decoction

治心氣不足，吐血衄血者，此湯主之。

A treatment for insufficiency of heart qì, with blood ejection and nosebleed, this decoction rules it.

大黃（二兩）黃連黃芩（各一兩）

dà huáng	大黃	6g
huáng lián	黃連	3g
huáng qín	黃芩	3g

上三味，以水三升。煮取一升，頓服之。

Simmer the three ingredients above in 600ml of water until reduced to 200ml. Take in one single dose.

Song 歌曰:

火熱上攻心氣傷，
即云心氣不足。
清濁二道血洋洋，
火逼血從濁道出則為吐,
血從清道出則為衄血。
大黃二兩芩連一，
釜下抽薪請細詳。

Fire heat ascends and attacks and damages heart qì.
Namely referred as heart qì insufficiency.
The paths of the clear and turbid are both vast with blood.
Fire forces blood to flow from the path of the turbid, which results in [blood] ejection.
[When] blood flows from the path of the clear, there are nosebleeds.
Carefully ponder the method of drawing firewood from the cauldron below
by [using] six grams *dà huáng*, [and] three [each] of *huáng qín* and [*huáng*] *lián.*

Commentary by Wèi 蔚按:

火邪盛而迫血，則錯經妄行。血為心液，血傷無以養心，致心陰之氣不足也，故曰心氣不足，非心陽之氣不足也。用芩、連苦寒之品，入心清火以培心氣；大黄去瘀生新，此一補一瀉之法也。

[When] fire evil is exuberant and distresses the blood this leads to derangement of the channels with frenetic movement. Blood is the humor of the heart, and when damaged, fails to nourish it, resulting in an insufficiency of the qì of heart yīn. Therefore, this is called insufficiency of the heart qì, and not insufficiency of the qì of heart yáng. Bitter and cold medicinals *huáng qín* and *huáng lián* enter the heart and clear fire in order to bank up heart qì; *dà huáng* eliminates stasis and engenders the new. This is a method [of treatment] in which [both] supplementation and drainage are used.

嘔吐噦下利方

Ǒu Tù Yuě Xià Lì Fāng

Formulas for Retching, Hiccup, and Diarrhea

吴茱萸湯

Wú Zhū Yú Tāng

Evodia Decoction

歌見《傷寒》。

For the song, see the *Shāng Hán Lùn.*

治嘔而胸滿者。

A treatment for retching and chest fullness.

吴茱萸（一升）人參（三兩）生薑（六兩）大棗（十二枚）

wú zhū yú	吴茱萸	200ml
rén shēn	人參	9g
shēng jiāng	生薑	18g
dà zǎo	大棗	12 pcs

上四味，以水五升，煮取三升，溫服七合，日三服。

Simmer the four ingredients above in 1,000ml of water until reduced to 600ml. Take 140ml warm, three doses per day.

又主乾嘔、吐涎沫、頭痛者。

Also rules [the treatment] of dry retching, vomiting of drool and spittle, and headaches.

Commentary by Lín Lǐfēng 受業林禮豐按:

胸為陽位，曠若太空，嘔而胸滿者，陰邪佔居陽位也，故重用生薑、吳萸之大辛大溫，以通胸中之陽，以破陰霾之氣；佐以人參、大棗之一陰一陽，以健脾胃之氣，以鎮逆上陰，使陽光普照，而陰翳自消，有何乾嘔、胸滿、涎沫之患哉？

The chest is the location of yáng, which is vast like the sky. With retching and chest fullness, yīn evil has occupied the position of yáng. Therefore, large doses of the majorly acrid and warm *shēng jiāng* and *wú zhū yú* are used in order to free yáng within the chest, and break the haze of qì. The assistants *rén shēn* and *dà zǎo,* one being yīn the other yáng, fortify spleen and stomach qì in order to settle the counterflow of ascending yīn, enabling the sunlight to illuminate everything, which will result in the dispersion of concealed yīn on its own. How [then] could there be any [more] trouble with dry retching, chest fullness, and drool and spittle?

半夏瀉心湯

Bàn Xià Xiè Xīn Tāng

Pinellia Heart-Draining Decoction

歌見《傷寒》。

For the song, see the *Shāng Hán Lùn.*

治嘔而腸鳴，心下痞者，此湯主之。

A treatment for retching with intestinal rumbling, and glomus below the heart, this decoction rules it.

半夏（半升，洗）黄芩（三兩）乾薑（三兩）人參（三兩）黄連（一兩）大棗（十二枚）甘草（三兩，炙）

bàn xià	半夏	washed	100ml
huáng qín	黄芩		9g
gān jiāng	乾薑		9g
rén shēn	人參		9g
huáng lián	黄連		3g
dà zǎo	大棗		12 pcs
gān cǎo	甘草	honey-fried	9g

上七味，以水一斗，煮取六升，去滓，再取三升，溫服一升，日三服。

Simmer the seven ingredients above in 2,000ml of water until reduced to 1,200ml. Remove the dregs and simmer again until reduced to 600ml. Take 200ml warm, three doses per day.

Commentary by eldest son [Chén] Wèi 長男蔚按:

嘔而腸鳴並無下利，心下痞不因誤下，何以上下之阻隔若是？蓋因飲停心下，上逆爲嘔，下乾爲腸鳴，飲不除則痞不消，欲蠲飲必資中氣。方中參、棗、草以培中氣，藉半夏之降逆，佐芩、連以消痞，複得乾薑之溫散，使痞者通，逆者降矣。妙在去滓再煎，取其輕清上浮，以成化痞降逆之用耳。

[When] retching and intestinal rumbling [occur] simultaneously without diarrhea, and [there is] glomus below the heart, which is not the result of erroneous precipitation, then why is there separation between the upper and lower? The reason is that rheum has collected below the heart, resulting in upward counterflow with retching, and disturbance of the lower with intestinal rumbling. [If] rheum is not eliminated, then the glomus will not disperse. [If one] desires to eliminate rheum, [one] must support the qì of the center. Within the formula, ***rén shēn, dà zǎo,*** and ***gān cǎo*** are used to bank up central qì, and ***bàn xià's*** [function] of downbearing counterflow is [also] utilized; the assistants ***huáng qín*** and ***huáng lián*** are used to disperse glomus, and in conjunction with warm and acrid *gān jiāng*, glomus is freed and counterflow is brought down. The ingenuity lies in the [method] of boiling the decoction again after removing the dregs, [making it] light and clear [which affects] the upper, [and] is able to transform glomus and downbear counterflow.

黄芩加半夏生薑湯

Huáng Qín Jiā Bàn Xià Shēng Jiāng Tāng

Scutellaria Decoction plus Pinellia and Fresh Ginger

歌見《傷寒》。

For the song, see the *Shāng Hán Lùn*.

治乾嘔而利者，此湯主之 。

A treatment for dry retching and diarrhea, this decoction rules it.

黄芩（ 三兩 ）甘草（ 二兩，炙 ）芍藥（ 二兩 ）半夏（ 半升 ）生薑（ 三兩 ）大棗（ 十二枚 ）

huáng qín	黄芩		9g
gān cǎo	甘草	honey-fried	6g
sháo yào	芍藥		6g
bàn xià	半夏		100ml
shēng jiāng	生薑		9g
dà zǎo	大棗		12 pcs

上六味，以水一斗，煮取三升，去滓 、溫服一升，日再夜一服 。

Simmer the six ingredients above in 2,000ml of water until reduced to 600ml. Remove the dregs and take 200ml warm, once during the day and again at night.

Commentary by [Chén] Yuánxī 男元犀按：

太陽主開，少陽主樞。乾嘔者，少陽之邪欲從太陽之開而外出也。下利者，太陽之邪不能從樞外出而反從樞內陷也。用黄芩加半夏生薑湯者，轉少陽之樞，達太陽之氣，交上下，清裏熱，而薑、夏又能止嘔降逆也。此即小柴胡湯去柴胡、人參加芍藥，去之者，恐其助飲而增嘔；加之者，取其和胃而降逆。伊聖之方，鬼神莫測也！

Tàiyáng rules opening, and shàoyáng rules the pivot. With dry retching, evil in shàoyáng desires to leave from the opening of tàiyáng. With diarrhea, tàiyáng evil is unable to exit outwards through the pivot, and instead sinks inwards. *Huáng Qín Jiā Bàn Xià Shēng Jiāng Tāng* is used to restore the pivot of shàoyáng and outthrust the qì of tàiyáng to [promote the] interaction of the upper and lower, and clear interior heat. *Shēng jiāng* and *bàn xià* can also stop retching and downbear counterflow. This [formula] is *Xiǎo Chái Hú Tāng* with *chái hú* and *rén shēn* removed and *sháo yào* added. [These medicinals] are removed out of fear of assisting rheum and increasing the retching. [*Sháo yào*] is added to harmonize the stomach and downbear counterflow. This is a formula of Master Yī's,[72] [whose] spirit [was] too profound to be understood.

72. Referring to Yī Yǐn 伊尹 the compiler of the *Tāng Yè Jīng* 《湯液經》(Decoction Classic), from which this formula originates.

小半夏湯

Xiǎo Bàn Xià Tāng

Minor Pinellia Decoction

治諸嘔吐，谷不得下者，此湯主之 。

A treatment for various kinds of vomiting, where food is unable to be taken, this decoction rules it.

半夏（ 一升 ）生薑（ 半斤 ）

bàn xià	半夏	200ml
shēng jiāng	生薑	24g

上二味，以水七升，煮取一升半，分溫再服 。

Simmer the two ingredients above in 1,400ml of water until reduced to 300ml. Divide and take warm in two doses.

Commentary by [Chén Yuán] Xī 犀按:

胃主納谷，谷不得下者，胃氣虛寒也。嘔吐者，飲隨寒氣上逆也，胃虛飲逆，非溫不能散其寒，非新[73]不能降其逆。用半夏滌飲降逆，生薑溫中散寒，使胃氣溫和，而嘔吐自平。

The stomach rules the intake of grains, [and if] there is an inability to get grain down it is [due] to stomach qì vacuity cold. Vomiting [is the result of] ascending counterflow of rheum, [which] follows cold qì. [With] stomach vacuity [there is] counterflow rheum. Without [the use of] warm [medicinals] cold would be unable to be dispersed, and without [the use of] acrid [medicinals], counterflow would be unable to be brought down. [Therefore] *bān xià* is used to flush rheum and downbear counterflow; *shēng jiāng* warms the center and dissipates cold, causing warmth and harmony of stomach qì, so the vomiting can be calmed on its own.

73. I believe that the character here 新 is a typographical error, and should actually be 辛, which means acrid. Both characters are pronounced as *xīn*.

豬苓散

Zhū Líng Sǎn

Polyporus Powder

治嘔吐而病在膈上，後思水者，解，急與之；思水者，此散主之。

[When] treating vomiting from diseases above the diaphragm, where [the vomiting] is followed by a desire for water, [this means] the disease will resolve, and [one should] immediately give [the patient] water. [If] there is a desire for water, this powder rules it.

豬苓茯苓白朮（各等分）

zhū líng	豬苓	equal parts of each ingredient
fú líng	茯苓	
bái zhú	白朮	

上三味，杵為散，飲服方寸匕，日三服。

Process the three ingredients above by pestling into a powder, and take one gram in fluid, three doses per day.

Song 歌曰:

嘔餘思水與之佳，
少與之飲，以救其液。
過與須防飲氣乖，
恐舊飲方去，新飲復來。
豬朮茯苓等分搗，
崇土以逐水，不使
支飲阻其正津，則不渴。
飲調寸匕自和諧。

After [one] vomits [and has] a desire for water, it is good to supply [water].
Give a small amount to drink in order to save the fluids.

Excessive amounts [are avoided] so as to avoid the return of counterflow rheum qì.
For fear of new rheum returning [following] the elimination of old rheum.
Pound equal parts of *zhū líng, bái zhú,* and *fú líng* with a pestle,
[In order to] support [the] earth and expel water, so as to not cause
propping-rheum [with] obstruction of right liquids, as a result [there is] no thirst.
A gram [of powder] mixed with fluid [will bring forth] spontaneous harmony.

四逆湯

Sì Nì Tāng

Frigid Extremities Decoction

歌見《傷寒》。

For the song, see the *Shāng Hán Lùn*.

治嘔而脈弱，小便復利，身有微熱，見厥者難治，此湯主之。

[When] treating retching with a weak pulse, uninhibited urination, and slight heat effusion in the body, [if] reversal is [seen], it is hard to treat, and this decoction rules it.

附子（一枚，生用）乾薑（一兩半）甘草（二兩，炙）

fù zǐ	附子	raw	1 pc
gān jiāng	乾薑		4.5g
gān cǎo	甘草	honey-fried	6g

上三味，以水三升，煮取一升二合，去滓，分溫再服。強人可大附子一枚，乾薑三兩。

Simmer the three ingredients above in 600ml of water until reduced to 140ml. Remove the dregs and take warm in two doses. For strong patients, one large piece of *fù zǐ* and nine grams of *gān jiāng* can be used.

Commentary by [Chén] Yuánxī 男元犀按：

嘔與熱為陰邪所迫，小便利與見厥，證屬無陽。脈弱者，真臟虛寒也。用四逆湯徹上下之陰邪，招欲散之殘陽，引氣血接回其厥，外溫經，內溫臟，面面俱到。

[Here, the] retching and heat are due to distress caused by yīn evil. [When] there is uninhibited urination presenting with reversal, this is a pattern of absence of yáng. A weak pulse signifies that there is true visceral vacuity cold. *Sì Nì Tāng* is used to penetrate the yīn evil in the upper and lower, attend to the dissipation of damaged yáng, facilitate the reconnection of [both] qì and blood, and stem reversal. By warming the channels on the exterior and the viscera in the interior, the entire situation is handled.

小柴胡湯

Xiǎo Chái Hú Tāng

Minor Bupleurum Decoction

歌見《傷寒》。

For the song, see the *Shāng Hán Lùn*.

治嘔而發熱者，此湯主之。

A treatment for retching and heat effusion, this decoction rules it.

柴胡（半斤）黃芩（三兩）人參（三兩）甘草（三兩）半夏（半斤）生薑（三兩）大棗（十二枚）

chái hú	柴胡	24g
huáng qín	黃芩	9g
rén shēn	人參	9g
gān cǎo	甘草	9g
bàn xià	半夏	24g
shēng jiāng	生薑	9g
dà zǎo	大棗	12 pcs

上七味，以水一斗二升，煮取六升，去滓，再煎取三升，溫服一升，日三服。

Simmer the seven ingredients above in 2,400ml of water until reduced to 1,200ml. Remove the dregs and simmer again until reduced to 600ml. Take 200ml warm, three doses per day.

Commentary by [Chén] Wèi 男蔚按：

嘔而發熱者，少陽表症也。表未解則內不和，故作嘔也。陽明主肌肉，木邪忤土，故作肌熱而嘔。用小柴胡湯轉樞以出其邪，邪解則熱退而嘔止也。

Retching and heat effusion are [due to] a shàoyáng exterior pattern. The exterior has not yet been resolved and the interior is not harmonized, leading to retching. Yángmíng governs the muscles and flesh, and when wood evil is hostile towards the earth, this results in heat in the flesh and retching. *Xiǎo Chái Hú Tāng* is used to shift the pivot in order to expel the evil, and when the evil has resolved then heat will abate and the retching will stop.

大半夏湯

Dà Bàn Xià Tāng

Major Pinellia Decoction

治胃反嘔吐者，此湯主之。

A treatment for stomach reflux and vomiting, this decoction rules it.

半夏（ 二升 ）人參（ 三兩 ）白蜜（ 一升 ）

bàn xià	半夏	400ml
rén shēn	人參	9g
bái mì	白蜜	200ml

上三味，水一斗二升，和蜜揚之二百四十遍，煮藥，取二升半，溫服一升，餘分再服。

Add the three ingredients above to 2,400ml of water, combine with honey, stir 240 times, and simmer until reduced to 500ml. Take 200ml warm, and take the rest in two doses.

Song 歌曰:

從來胃反責之衝脈上乘，
半夏二升蜜一升，
三兩人參勞水煮，
水揚二百四十遍
名勞水，又名甘瀾水。
納衝養液有奇能。

Whenever [there is] stomach reflux, blame the **upward** ascension of the thoroughfare **vessel**.
400ml of *bàn xià*, 200ml of honey,
and nine grams of *rén shēn*, boiled in worked water,[74]
water that has been stirred two hundred and forty times

74. The term "worked water" first appears in the *Huáng Dì Nèi Jīng*.

is called worked water, or *gān lán shǔi*,
has the special ability of absorbing the surging, and nourishing the fluids.

Commentary by [Chén] Yuánxī 元犀按:

此方用水之多，取其多煮白蜜，去其寒而用其潤，俾粘膩之性流連於胃。不速下行；而半夏、人參之力，可以徐徐斡旋於中。非參透造化之理者，不能悟及。余遇醫輩偶談及於此，不能再三問難，便知其庸陋欺人，則不復與談矣。

This formula uses copious amounts of water so that the honey can be simmered for an extended period of time in order to remove [the honey's] coldness and utilize its moistening [function]. This enables the sticky and slimy nature to remain within the stomach, avoiding downward movement [from occurring] too quickly; [this way] the strength of *bàn xià* and *rén shēn* can gently mediate the center. Unless one thoroughly understands the creators' theory, one cannot comprehend this! I occasionally speak of this with physicians I encounter. [If these physicians] are unable to discuss this [difficulty] in more depth, I would know that they are inferior, limited [physicians who are] deceiving people, and [I] then no longer [continue to] discuss it [with them].

膈咽之間，交通之氣不得降者，皆冲脉上行，逆氣所作也。師以半夏降衝脈之逆，即以白蜜潤陽明之燥，加人參以生既亡之津液，用甘瀾水以降逆上之水液。古聖之經方，惟師能用之。

[The reason] the interaction of qì between the throat and diaphragm is unable to descend, [is due to] the upward movement of the thoroughfare vessel, [which] is regarded as counterflow qì. The master used *bàn xià* to downbear counterflow in the thoroughfare vessel, and honey to moisten the dryness of yángmíng. *Rén shēn* is added to generate the already collapsed fluids, and worked water is utilized to downbear [the] counterflow of water liquids. This is an ancient and sacred classical formula, which only a master [Zhòngjǐng] could use.

大黄甘草湯
Dà Huáng Gān Cǎo Tāng
Rhubarb and Licorice Decoction

治食已即吐者，此湯主之。

A treatment for vomiting immediately after eating, this decoction rules it.

大黄（四兩）甘草（二兩）

dà huáng	大黄	12g
gān cǎo	甘草	6g

上二味，以水三升，煮取一升，分溫再服。

Simmer the two ingredients above in 600ml of water until reduced to 200ml. Divide and take warm in two doses.

Song 歌曰：

食方未久吐相隨，食已即吐。
兩熱衝來自不支；
胃素有熱，食復入之，
兩熱相衝，不停片刻而吐出。
四兩大黄二兩草，
上從下取法神奇。

Vomiting not long following a meal, **vomiting immediately after eating,**
[is the result of] two kinds of heat [which are] surging, and are difficult to endure.
[When] there is heat in the stomach, and [hot-natured] food enters,
the two kinds of heat surge [upwards, food is] not lodged and vomit issues a moment later.
Twelve grams of *dà huáng* and six of *gān cǎo* offer a marvelous method
[in which] the ascending [counterflow is brought down] by following precipitation.

Commentary by [Chén] Wèi 蔚按:

師云：欲吐者，不可下之。又云：食已即吐者，大黃甘草湯下之。二說相反，何也？曰：病在上而欲吐，宜因而越之；若逆之使下，則憒亂矣；若既吐矣，吐而不已，是有升無降，當逆折之。

The master said that with a desire to vomit, [one] cannot cause precipitation. He also said that with vomiting immediately after eating, [use] *Dà Huáng Gān Cǎo Tāng* to precipitate it. How is it that he can say two contrary things? It is said that when disease is in the upper, and there is a desire to vomit, it should be brought up and out [yet] if on the contrary it is brought down, then this will bring forth trouble and disorder! If there is already vomiting, and ejection [therapy] has been used, [and the vomiting] has not ceased, we [know] there is upbearing and no downbearing, [and this] counterflow must be reversed.

Quotation by Yóu Zàijīng 尤在涇云:

雲霧出於地，而雨露降於天，地不承則天不降矣。可見天地陰陽同此氣機，和則俱和，乖則並乖。人與天地相參，故肺氣象天，病則多及二陰；脾、胃、大小腸象地，病則多及上竅。丹溪治小便不通，用吐法而升提肺氣，使上竅開而下竅亦通，與大黃甘草湯之治嘔吐，法雖異而理可通也。

Clouds and mist emit from the earth, and rain and dew descend from the heavens. [If] the earth cannot comply then the heavens cannot descend. It can be clearly seen that when heaven and earth and yīn and yáng are in harmony together with the qì mechanism, all will be harmonious, and if disharmonious, all will be in disharmony. There is a similarity between people and heaven and earth. Lung qì resembles heaven, and when diseased, will commonly reach [and affect] the two [lower] yīn; the spleen, stomach, and large and small intestines resemble the earth, and when diseased will commonly reach [and affect] the upper orifices. Zhū Dānxī[75] treated inhibited urination by using a method of ejection to raise lung qì, causing the opening of the upper orifices to free the lower orifices. This [particular method] is similar to the use of *Dà Huáng Gān Cǎo Tāng* for treating vomiting, and although these methods are different, their theories [and outcomes] are the same.

75. Zhū Dānxī was a famous scholar and physician of the *Jīn Yuán* Dynasty.

茯苓澤瀉湯

Fú Líng Zé Xiè Tāng

Poria and Alisma Decoction

治胃反，吐而渴欲飲水者，此湯主之。

A treatment for stomach reflux with thirst and a desire to drink water following vomiting, this decoction rules it.

茯苓（半斤）澤瀉（四兩）甘草桂枝（各二兩）白朮（三兩）生薑（四兩）

fú líng	茯苓	24g
zé xiè	澤瀉	12g
gān cǎo	甘草	6g
guì zhī	桂枝	6g
bái zhú	白朮	9g
shēng jiāng	生薑	12g

上六味，以水一斗，煮取三升，內澤瀉，再煮取二升半，溫服八合，日三服。

Simmer the five ingredients above [without the *zé xiè*] in 2,000ml of water until reduced to 600ml. Add the *zé xiè*, and simmer again until reduced to 500ml. Take 160ml warm, three doses per day.

《外臺》治消渴脈絕胃反者，有小麥一升。

The *Wài Tái Mì Yào* says to treat dispersion thirst with an expiring pulse and stomach reflux, add 200ml of *xiāo mài*.

Song 歌曰:

吐方未已渴頻加，
與吐後渴為欲愈者不同，
亦與豬苓散症未吐而先渴者不同。
苓八兩生薑四兩誇，
二兩桂甘三兩朮，
澤須四兩後煎嘉。
後煮澤瀉，取其補陰而利水，
不宜煮之太過也。

Vomiting has not yet ceased [and there is] frequent thirst [which has] increased.
This is different than the thirst following vomiting which indicates imminent recovery,
and is also different than the *Zhū Líng Săn* pattern of thirst before any vomiting.
Twenty-four grams of *fú líng* and twelve of *shēng jiāng* is great;
six grams of *guì zhī* and *gān căo* with nine of *bái zhú.*
Afterwards, adding twelve grams of *zé xiè* and simmering is excellent.
Adding *zé xiè* after boiling obtains the yīn supplementing and water disinhibiting [effects],
for it is inappropriate to boil it excessively.

Quotation by Xú Zhōngkě 徐忠可云:

此方於五苓散中去豬苓者，以胃反證，水從吐出，中無水氣而渴也；加生薑、甘草者，合苓、朮等藥以解表裏之虛邪，更能和中而止嘔也。

With this formula, the reason *zhū líng* is removed from *Wŭ Líng Săn* is that there is stomach reflux, and [since] water follows vomit outwards, [this] leaves the center without water qì, resulting in thirst. *Shēng jiāng* and *gān căo* are added, and in combination with *fú líng, bái zhú* and the other medicinals are able to resolve vacuous evils in the exterior and interior, [thereby] harmonizing the center and stopping the vomiting.

文蛤湯

Wén Gé Tāng

Clamshell Decoction

治吐後渴欲得水而貪飲者，此湯主之；兼主微風、脈緊、頭痛。

A treatment for thirst with a desire for water and voracious drinking after vomiting, this decoction rules it. It simultaneously rules [the treatment of] mild wind [with a] tight pulse, and headaches.

文蛤石膏（各五兩）麻黄甘草生薑（各三兩）杏仁（五十粒）大棗（十二枚）

wén gé	文蛤	15g
shí gāo	石膏	15g
má huáng	麻黄	9g
gān cǎo	甘草	9g
shēng jiāng	生薑	9g
xìng rén	杏仁	50 kernels
dà zǎo	大棗	12 pcs

上七味，以水六升，煮取二升，溫服一升，汗出即愈。

Simmer the seven ingredients above in 1,200ml of water until reduced to 400ml. Take 200ml warm. Sweating [indicates] immediate recovery.

Song 歌曰:

吐而貪飲證宜詳，
文蛤石膏五兩量，
十二棗枚杏五十，
麻甘三兩等生薑。

A pattern of vomiting with a voracious desire to drink fluids should [be dealt with] carefully.
[Use] fifteen grams of *wén gé* and *shí gāo,*

twelve pieces of *dà zǎo*, and fifty of *xìng rén*,
[with] nine grams each *má huáng*, *gān cǎo* and *shēng jiāng*.

Commentary by [Chén] Yuánxī 元犀按:

水雖隨吐而去，而熱不與水俱去，故貪飲不休，與思水者不同。方中麻黄與石膏並用，能深入伏熱之中，頃刻透出於外，從汗而解，熱解則渴亦解，故不用止渴之品。並主微風、脈緊、頭痛者，以風爲陽邪，得此涼散之劑而恰對也。

Although water is expelled with vomiting, heat is not eliminated with the water; so therefore there is incessant, voracious drinking of fluids, which is not the same as a desire for fluids. In the formula, *má huáng* and *shí gāo* are used together for their ability to penetrate into deep-lying heat, and instantly outthrust it into the exterior, to be resolved through sweat. When heat is resolved, thirst will also be abated. It is for this reason that medicinals which allay thirst are not used. [It also] simultaneously rules [the treatment of] mild wind, [with a] tight pulse, and headache. Wind is a yáng evil, and when this cooling powder formula is taken, it can [be] properly opposed.

半夏乾薑散
Bàn Xià Gān Jiāng Sǎn
Pinellia and Dried Ginger Powder

治乾嘔吐逆，吐涎沫者，此散主之 。

A treatment for dry retching, vomiting counterflow, and vomiting of drool and spittle, this powder rules it.

半夏乾薑（ 各等分 ）

bàn xià	半夏	equals amounts of each ingredient
gān jiāng	乾薑	

上二味，杵為散，取方寸匕，漿水一升半，煮取七合，頓服之 。

Pestle [equal parts of] the two ingredients above into a powder, and simmer one gram with 300ml of sour millet water until reduced to 140ml. Take in a single dose.

Song 歌曰:

吐而乾嘔沫涎多，
惟不胸滿，不頭痛，
與吳茱萸湯證不同。
以虛有微甚，邪有高下之別也。
胃腑不責於厥陰，專責於陽明。
虛寒氣不和，
薑夏等分磨漿水煮，
數方小半夏湯、生薑半夏湯。
相類頗分科 。漿水甘酸，
能調中引氣，止嘔噦。

Vomiting and dry retching with copious drool and spittle.
This is different than a *Wú Zhū Yú Tāng* pattern, as there is no chest fullness or headaches;

the vacuity is slight [in this formula], and prominent [in a *Wú Zhū Yú Tāng* pattern], while [the location of] the evil is higher as opposed to lower.
The stomach bowel **is not controlled by juéyīn, [but is] specifically controlled by yángmíng,** [suffers from] vacuity cold qì disharmony,
[use] equal parts *bàn xià* and *shēng jiāng* ground and boiled with sour millet water.
Several [other] formulas, **[such as] *Xiǎo Bàn Xià Tāng* and *Shēng Jiāng Bàn Xià Tāng*,** are similar but not the same. **Sour millet water is both sweet and sour, which can regulate the center, lead qì [downwards], and stop retching.**

生薑半夏湯

Shēng Jiāng Bàn Xià Tāng

Fresh Ginger and Pinellia Decoction

治病人胸中似喘不喘，似嘔不嘔，似噦不噦，徹心中憒憒無奈者，此湯主之。

A treatment for patients who feel a [sensation] in the chest of panting but do not pant, a [sensation of] retching, but do not retch, a [sensation of] hiccuping but do not hiccup, and heart fretting with helplessness, this decoction rules it.

半夏（ 半升 ）生薑（ 汁，一升 ）

bàn xià	半夏		100ml
shēng jiāng	生薑	juice	200ml

上二味，以水三升，煮半夏，取二升，內生薑汁，煮取一升半，小冷，分四服，日三夜一，嘔止，停後服 。

Use 600ml of water for the two ingredients above, first simmering the *bàn xià*, until reduced to 400ml. Add the *shēng jiāng* juice and simmer until reduced to 300ml. [When] it is slightly cool, divide into four doses, and take three throughout the day, and one at night. When the vomiting has stopped, discontinue use.

Song 歌曰:

嘔噦都非喘又非，
似嘔之狀，不似嘔之有物；
似噦之有聲，不似噦之連聲；
似喘之氣逆，不似喘之氣急。
徹心憒憒莫從違；
懊憹之甚，無可奈何，
皆飲邪與寒邪搏結於胸。
一升薑汁半升夏，
分煮同煎妙入微 。

Retching and hiccups [are] both absent, as is panting.
[This is] similar to retching, but not like retching with matter;
resembles hiccups with sound, but sound does not repeat;
resembles the counterflow qì of panting, but is not like the rapid breathing of panting.
Heart fretting with helplessness, where one does not know what to do.
When anguish is severe, [one] is utterly helpless,
[which is due to] the uniting and binding of rheum and cold evils in the chest.
200ml of *shēng jiāng* juice, with 100ml of *bàn xià* separately simmered,
and [then] boiled together is ingenious in every possible way.

Comparison 參:

與吳茱萸之降濁、乾薑之溫中不同。蓋彼乃虛寒上逆，此乃客邪搏飲也。方即小半夏湯，不用薑而用汁者，以降逆之力少，散結之力多也。

The turbidity downbearing [effect] of *wú zhū yú* is different than *gān jiāng's* ability to warm the center, as *wú zhū yú* is [used] for vacuity cold with ascending counterflow, and *gān jiāng* is [used] for visiting evil contending with rheum. This formula is *Xĭao Bàn Xià Tāng* [but] with the juice of *shēng jiāng* being used instead of the root, as its ability to downbear counterflow is quite weak, while its ability to disperse binds is quite strong.

橘皮湯
Jú Pí Tāng
Tangerine Peel Decoction

治乾嘔噦，若手足厥者，此湯主之。

A treatment for dry retching with hiccups, [where] if there is reversal of the extremities, this decoction rules it.

橘皮（四兩）生薑（半斤）

jú pí	橘皮	12g
shēng jiāng	生薑	24g

上二味，以水七升，煮取三升，溫服一升，下咽即愈。

Simmer the two ingredients above in 1,400ml of water until reduced to 600ml, and take 200ml warm. There will be resolution once it is swallowed.

Song 歌曰:

噦而乾嘔厥相隨。
氣逆於胸阻四肢；
乾嘔非胃反，厥非無陽，
乃氣逆於胸，不行於四末故也。
初病未虛一服驗，
生薑八兩四陳皮。

Hiccups, dry retching, and reversal are all [present] together.
Counterflow qì in the chest obstructs the extremities.
[This is] dry retching and not stomach reflux. This reversal is not [due to] an absence of yáng, but to counterflow qì in the chest causing lack of movement in the extremities.
At the onset of the disease there is no vacuity, and one dose
of twenty-four grams of *shēng jiāng* and twelve of *chén pí* should prove effective.

Commentary by [Chén] Yuánxī 元犀按:

《金匱》論噦，與方書不同，專指呃逆而言也。

The *Jīn Guì Yào Lüè's* discussion on hiccups is quite different than [various] other formula books. The *Jīn Guì Yào Lüè* specifically refers to it as hiccup counterflow.[76]

76. The *Jīn Guì Yào Lüè* always used the character *yuě* 噦 when discussing hiccups.

橘皮竹茹湯
Jú Pí Zhú Rú Tāng
Tangerine Peel and Bamboo Shavings Decoction

治噦逆者，此湯主之。

A treatment for hiccup counterflow, this decoction rules it.

橘皮（ 二斤 ）竹茹（ 二斤 ）大棗（ 三十枚 ）生薑（ 半斤 ）甘草（ 五兩 ）人參（ 一兩 ）

jú pí	橘皮	96g
zhú rú	竹茹	96g
dà zǎo	大棗	30 pcs
shēng jiāng	生薑	24g
gān cǎo	甘草	15g
rén shēn	人參	3g

上六味，以水一斗，煮取三升，溫服一升，日三服。

Simmer the six ingredients above in 2,000ml of water until reduced to 600ml. Take 200ml warm, three doses per day.

Song 歌曰:

噦逆因虛熱氣乘，
一參五草八薑勝，
棗枚三十二斤橘，
生竹青皮即竹茹也。刮二升。

Hiccup counterflow is caused by heat qì overwhelming vacuity;
three grams of *rén shēn,* fifteen grams of *gān cǎo,* and twenty-four of *shēng jiāng* will prevail.
[Combine with] thirty-pieces of *dà zǎo,* ninety-six grams of *jú pí,*
and 400ml of scraped *shēng zhú qīng pí* **namely *zhú rú.***

Commentary by [Chén Yuán] Xī 犀按:

《淺注》已詳方義，不再釋。《金匱》以呃為噦，凡呃逆證，皆是寒熱错亂，二氣相搏使然。故方中用生薑、竹茹，一寒一熱以祛之；人參、橘皮，一開一合以分之；甘草、大棗奠安中土，使中土有權，而噦逆自平矣。此伊聖經方，扁鵲丁香柿蒂散即從此方套出也。

The *Jīn Guì Yào Lüè Qiǎn Zhù*[77] already gives a detailed explanation of the formula, so there is no need to explain again. The *Jīn Guì Yào Lüè* [always] used the character *yuě* 噦 for *è* 呃, which both mean hiccup, and considered it to be a complex disorder resulting from the contention of cold and heat qì. Therefore, the formula uses *shēng jiāng* and *zhú rú*, one hot and one cold medicinal, in order to dispel the cold and heat qì, and *rén shēn* and *jú pí*, one opening and one closing medicinal, in order to separate [counterflow]. *Gān cǎo* and *dà zǎo* settle and quiet central earth, creating a powerful center earth so hiccups and counterflow are naturally calmed. This is Master Yī's classical formula, from which Biǎn Què's *Dīng Xiāng Shì Dì Sǎn* is modeled.

77. The Shallow Commentary on the *Jīn Guì Yào Lüè*, written by Chén Xiūyuán ca. 1820 in ten scrolls.

四逆湯

Sì Nì Tāng

Frigid Extremities Decoction

歌解見《傷寒》。

For the song with explanation, see the *Shāng Hán Lùn*.

治下利後，腹脹滿，身體疼痛者，先溫其裏，乃攻其表。溫裏宜四逆湯，攻表宜桂枝湯。

A treatment for abdominal distention and fullness, and generalized pain following diarrhea; first one must warm the interior, and then attack the exterior. To warm the interior, *Sì Nì Tāng* is appropriate, and to attack the exterior give *Guì Zhī Tāng*.

桂枝湯

Guì Zhī Tāng

Cinnamon Twig Decoction

歌解見《傷寒》。

For the song with explanation, see the *Shāng Hán Lùn.*

桂枝（ 三兩，去皮 ）芍藥（ 三兩 ）甘草（ 二兩，炙 ）生薑（ 三兩 ）大棗（ 十二枚 ）

guì zhī	桂枝	bark removed	9g
sháo yào	芍藥		9g
gān cǎo	甘草	honey-fried	6g
shēng jiāng	生薑		9g
dà zǎo	大棗		12 pcs

上五味，㕮咀，以水七升，微火煮取三升，去滓，適寒溫服一升，服已須臾，啜稀粥一升，以助藥力，溫覆令一時許，遍身漐漐微似有汗者、益佳，不可令如水淋漓，若一服汗出病瘥，停後服。

Break the five ingredients above into small pieces, and simmer over a mild flame in 1,400ml of water until reduced to 600ml. Remove the dregs and take 200ml at moderate temperature. Shortly after, drink 100ml of hot, thin gruel in order to reinforce the strength of the medicinals. Warm the body by covering up [with a blanket] for a short period, until the whole body is moist as if sweating very lightly. One cannot allow the sweat to pour like water. If one brings forth sweating, and the disease diminishes, stop taking further doses.

大承氣湯
Dà Chéng Qì Tāng
Major Qì Coordinating Decoction

歌解見《傷寒》。

For the song with explanation, see the *Shāng Hán Lùn*.

治下利，三部脈皆平，按之心下堅者，宜之。

A treatment for diarrhea, where all three-pulse positions are normal, and [with] hardness below the heart on palpation, [this formula] is appropriate.

治下利脈遲而滑者。實也；利未欲止，急下之，宜此湯。

A treatment for diarrhea with a slow and slippery pulse, [which signifies] an excess pattern, where the diarrhea is not yet on the verge of ceasing. This should be urgently precipitated, and this decoction is appropriate.

治下利脈反滑者，當有所去，下乃愈，宜此湯。

A treatment for diarrhea with an abnormally slippery pulse, which requires elimination. Precipitation will bring forth recovery, and this decoction is appropriate.

治下利已瘥，至其年月日時復發者，以病不盡故也，宜此湯。

A treatment for [after] the diarrhea has been resolved, it returns again at the same time as the initial onset; the reason is that the disease was never terminated. This decoction is appropriate.

大黃（四兩，酒洗）厚朴（半斤，炙，去皮）枳實（五枚）芒硝（三合）

dà huáng	大黃	washed in liquor	12g
hòu pò	厚朴	honey-fried and skin removed	24g
zhǐ shí	枳實		5 pcs
máng xiāo	芒硝		60ml

上四味，以水一斗，先煮二物，取五升，去滓，內大黃，煮取二升，去滓，內芒硝，更上火微一二沸，分溫再服，得下止服。

Of the four ingredients above, simmer the two substances [*zhǐ shí* and *hòu pò*] in 2,000ml of water until reduced to 1,000ml. Remove the dregs, add the *dà huáng*, and simmer until reduced to 400ml. Remove the dregs, add the *máng xiāo*, and again place it on a small flame to boil once or twice. Divide and take warm in two doses. As soon as precipitation [i.e., defecation] is achieved, stop taking it.

小承氣湯

Xiǎo Chéng Qì Tāng

Minor Qì Coordinating Decoction

歌解見《傷寒》。

For the song with explanation, see the *Shāng Hán Lùn*.

治下利譫語者，有燥屎也，宜此湯。

A treatment for diarrhea with delirious speech, [which indicates] dry stools, this decoction is appropriate.

大黃（四兩）厚朴（二兩，炙）枳實（大者三枚，炙）

dà huáng	大黃		12g
hòu pò	厚朴	honey-fried	6g
zhǐ shí	枳實	honey-fried	3 large pcs

上三味，以水四升，煮取一升二合，去滓，分溫二服，得利則止。

Simmer the three ingredients above in 800ml of water until reduced to 240ml. Remove the dregs, divide and take warm in two doses. Once diarrhea appears, the formula should be discontinued.

桃花湯

Táo Huā Tāng

Peach Blossom Decoction

歌解見《傷寒》。

For the song with explanation, see the *Shāng Hán Lùn*.

治下利便膿血者，宜此湯。

A treatment for diarrhea with pus and blood in the stools, this decoction is appropriate.

赤石脂（一斤，一半剉，一半篩末）乾薑（一兩）粳米（一升）

chì shí zhī	赤石脂	half shredded, half ground and sieved	48g
gān jiāng	乾薑		6g
jīng mǐ	粳米		200ml

上三味，以水七升，煮令米熟，去滓，溫服七合，內赤石脂末方寸匕，日三服。若一服愈，餘勿服。

Simmer the three ingredients above[78] in 1,400ml of water until the rice is fully cooked. Remove the dregs and take 140ml warm with one gram of powdered *chì shí zhī*, three doses per day. If the [disease] is cured after one dose, do not take the remainder [of the decoction].

78. While the cooking instructions are slightly unclear, it would be safe to assume that the shredded half of the *chì shí zhī* is cooked in the decoction, while the ground and sieved half is reserved, to be added to the decoction after it has been cooked.

白頭翁湯

Bái Tóu Wēng Tāng

Pulsatilla Decoction

歌解見《傷寒》。

For the song with explanation, see the *Shāng Hán Lùn*.

治熱利下重者，宜之。

A treatment for heat diarrhea with rectal heaviness [this formula] is appropriate.

白頭翁（二兩）黃連黃柏秦皮（各三兩）

bái tóu wēng	白頭翁	6g
huáng lián	黃連	9g
huáng bǎi	黃柏	9g
qín pí	秦皮	9g

上四味，以水七升，煮取二升、去滓、溫服一升、不愈，更服。

Simmer the four ingredients above in 1,400ml of water until reduced to 400ml. Remove the dregs and take 200ml warm. If there is no recovery, take another dose.

梔子豉湯

Zhī Zǐ Chǐ Tāng

Gardenia and Fermented Soybean Decoction

歌解見《傷寒》。

For the song with explanation, see the *Shāng Hán Lùn*.

治下利後更煩，按之心下濡者，為虛煩也，此主之 。

A treatment for [when] after diarrhea [there is] increased vexation, and sogginess below the heart when pressed. [This] indicates vacuity vexation, and this [formula] rules it.

梔子（ 十四枚 ）香豉（ 四合，綿裹 ）

zhī zǐ	梔子		14 pcs
xiāng chǐ	香豉	wrapped in gauze	80ml

上二味，以水四升，先煮梔子，得二升半，內豉，煮取一升半，去滓，分二服，溫進一服，得吐則止 。

Use 800ml of water for the two ingredients above. First simmer the *zhī zǐ* until reduced to 500ml, add the *xiāng chǐ*, and simmer until reduced to 300ml. Remove the dregs and divide into two doses. Stop taking if vomiting occurs.

通脈四逆湯

Tōng Mài Sì Nì Tāng

Channel Unblocking Frigid Extremities Decoction

歌解見《傷寒》。

For the song with explanation, see the *Shāng Hán Lùn*.

治下利清谷，裏寒外熱，汗出而厥，此主之。

A treatment for clear food diarrhea with interior cold and exterior heat with sweating and reversal, this [formula] rules it.

附子（大者一枚，生用）乾薑（三兩，強人可四兩）甘草（二兩，炙）

fù zǐ	附子	raw	1 large pc
gān jiāng	乾薑		9g (12g can be used for strong patients)
gān cǎo	甘草	honey-fried	6g

上三味，以水三升、煮取一升二合，去滓，分溫再服。

Simmer the three ingredients above in 600ml of water until reduced to 140ml. Remove the dregs. Divide and take warm in two doses.

紫參湯

Zǐ Shēn Tāng

Rhizoma Bistortae Decoction

治下利肺痛者，此湯主之 。

A treatment for diarrhea and lung pain, this decoction rules it.

紫參（ 半斤 ）甘草（ 三兩 ）

zǐ shēn	紫參	24g
gān cǎo	甘草	9g

上二味，以水五升，先煮紫參，取二升，內甘草，煮取一升半，分溫三服 。

Use 1,000ml of water for the two ingredients above. First simmer the *zǐ shēn* until the water is reduced to 400ml. Add the *gān cǎo* and simmer until reduced to 300ml. Divide and take warm in two doses.

Song 歌曰:

利而肺痛是何傷？
濁氣上乾責胃腸；
肺與大腸相表裏。
八兩紫參三兩草，
通因通用細推詳 。
腸中積聚，
是肺氣不行於大腸。

With diarrhea and lung pain, where is the damage?
The ascending assault of turbid qì is blamed on the stomach and intestines.
The lungs and the large intestine stand in interior and exterior relationship.
Carefully ponder [the method of] treating the free by freeing,
with twenty-four grams *zǐ shēn* and nine grams *gān cǎo*.
Lung qì is unable to move [descend] into the large intestine
due to the presence of accumulations and gatherings within the intestines.

Commentary by [Chén] Wèi 男蔚按：

肺為華蓋，諸臟之氣皆上熏之，惟胃腸之氣下降而不上乾於肺，故肺為清肅之臟而不受濁氣者也。夫肺與腸相表裏，腸胃相連，下利肺痛者，腸胃之濁氣上乾於肺也，故主以紫參湯。《本經》云：紫參主治心腹寒熱積聚邪氣；甘草解百毒，奠中土，使中土有權而肺金受益，腸胃通暢而肺氣自安，肺氣安則清肅之令行矣，何有肺痛下利之病哉？

The lungs are the florid canopy. The qì of all the viscera ascend and fume it. The qì of the stomach and intestines [should] descend [and] not ascend, [which can] assault the lungs. The lungs are the viscus of clearing and eliminating and should not receive turbid qì. The lungs and large intestine stand in an interior and exterior relationship, and the intestines and stomach are linked together. Diarrhea and lung pain are due to the ascent of turbid qì from the stomach and intestines, which assaults the lungs, and for this reason *Zǐ Shēn Tāng* rules. The *Shén Nóng Běn Cǎo Jīng* says that *zǐ shēn* rules the treatment of cold and heat accumulations and gatherings of evil qì in the heart and abdomen. *Gān cǎo* resolves the hundred toxins, and settles center earth enabling the power of center earth to benefit lung metal. When the intestines and stomach are unobstructed, lung qì will be calm by itself. [When] lung qì is calm, then its clearing and eliminating [function] will be carried out. How then could there be the disease of lung pain and diarrhea?

訶黎勒散

Hē Lí Lè Sǎn

Chebule Powder

治氣利者，此散主之 。

A treatment for qì diarrhea, this powder rules it.

訶黎勒（ 十枚 ）

hē lí lè 訶黎勒 10 pcs

上一味為散，粥飲和，頓服 。

Powder the ingredient above and take with rice gruel in one single dose.

Song 歌曰:

訶黎勒散澀腸便，
氣利還須固後天，
十個訶黎煨研末，
調和米飲不須煎 。

Hē Lí Lè Sǎn astringes the intestines,
[and with] qì diarrhea [one] must also secure later heaven.
Ten pieces of *hē lí lè* ground to a powder,
mixed with rice gruel; [there is] no need to decoct.

Commentary by [Chén] Yuánxī 男元犀按:

氣利者，肺氣下脫，胃腸俱虛，氣陷屎下。急用訶黎勒澀腸胃以固脫，又用粥飲扶中以轉氣，氣轉而瀉自止耳。

With qì diarrhea, [there is] lung qì desertion. [When] both the stomach and intestines are vacuous, [there is] sinking qì and descent of stools. Quickly use *Hē Lí Lè Săn* to astringe the intestines and stomach in order to secure desertion. Also use rice gruel to support the center in order to shift qì, as once qì has shifted, diarrhea will stop on its own.

附方
Fù Fāng
Attached Formulas

《千金翼》小承氣湯
Qiān Jīn Yì Xiǎo Chéng Qì Tāng

Minor Qì Coordinating Decoction from the *Qiān Jīn Yì*[79]

歌解見《傷寒》。

For the song with explanation, see the *Shāng Hán Lùn*.

治大便不通，噦數譫語。

A treatment for constipation, frequent hiccups and delirious speech.

79. This version of the formula is found in the Sudden Turmoil chapter of the book *Qiān Jīn Yì* 《千金翼》(Wings of the Thousand Gold Pieces Formulary) by Sūn Sīmiǎo and consists of *hòu pò* 6g, *dà huáng* 12g, and three large pieces of *zhǐ shí*, which is the same as found in the *Shāng Hán Lùn*.

《外臺》黄芩湯

Wài Tái Huáng Qín Tāng

Scutellaria Decoction from the *Wài Tái Mì Yào*

治乾嘔下利者。

A treatment for dry retching and diarrhea.

黄芩人參乾薑（各三兩）桂枝（一兩）大棗（十二枚）半夏（半升）

rén shēn	人參	9g
gān jiāng	乾薑	9g
guì zhī	桂枝	3g
dà zǎo	大棗	12 pcs
bàn xià	半夏	100ml

上六味，以水七升，煮取三升，溫分三服。

Simmer the six ingredients above in 1,400ml of water until reduced to 600ml. Divide and take warm in three doses.

Song 歌曰:

乾嘔利兮責二陽，
太陽陽明遞相傳也。
參芩三兩等乾薑，
桂枝一兩半升夏，
棗十二枚轉運良。

[With] dry retching and diarrhea, blame the two yángs.
Passage of tàiyáng to yángmíng.
Nine grams [each of] *rén shēn, huáng qín* and *gān jiāng;*
three grams *guì zhī,* 100ml *bàn xià,*
and twelve pieces of *dà zǎo* will bring forth [the] proper workings [of the qì dynamic].

Commentary by [Chén] Yuánxī 男元犀按:

此即小柴胡湯變法。方中以桂枝易柴胡，以乾薑易生薑，去甘草是也。太陽病不解，並入陽明，陰陽舛錯，而爲嘔吐下利也，方用黃芩、乾薑，寒温並进，使之入胃以分陰陽，又以参，枣安胃，桂枝祛邪，半夏降逆，且半夏生當夏半，正陰陽交界之間，取之以和陰陽。陰陽和則中樞轉，上下交而嘔利止矣。

This is a variant method of *Xiǎo Chái Hú Tāng*. In the formula, *chái hú* is replaced with *guì zhī*, *shēng jiāng* is replaced with *gān jiāng*, and *gān cǎo* is removed. When tàiyáng disease is unresolved, it will enter yángmíng, and yīn and yáng will be disordered[80] causing dry retching and diarrhea. The formula uses *huáng qín* and *gān jiāng*, one cold and one warm [medicinal] to advance together into the stomach in order to separate yīn and yáng. It also uses *rén shēn* and *dà zǎo* to calm the stomach, *guì zhī* to dispel evils, and *bàn xià* to downbear counterflow. Moreover, *bàn xià* grows in the midsummer between the border of yīn and yáng, so is [therefore] taken to harmonize yīn and yáng. When yīn and yáng are harmonized, then the central pivot shifts, the upper and lower interact, and the dry retching and diarrhea stop!

80. The characters *chuǎn cuò* 舛錯 are the equivilant of *cuò luàn* 錯亂, meaning "in disorder" or "deranged."

瘡癰腸癰浸淫病方

Chuāng Yōng Cháng Yōng Jìn Yín Bìng Fāng

Formulas for Sores, Welling-Abscess, Intestinal Welling-Abscess, and Wet and Spreading Sores

薏苡附子敗醬散

Yì Yǐ Fù Zǐ Bài Jiàng Sǎn

Coix, Aconite, and Patrinia Powder

治腸癰之為病，其身甲錯，腹皮急，按之濡，如腫狀，腹無積聚，身無熱，脈數，此為腸內有癰膿，此散主之。

A treatment for intestinal welling-abscess disease, with generalized skin encrustation, tense abdominal skin which is soggy on pressure and appears swollen, absence of abdominal accumulations and gatherings, no generalized heat, and rapid pulses. These [symptoms] indicate welling-abscess and pus in the intestines, and this powder rules it.

薏苡仁（十分）附子（二分）敗醬（五分）

yì yǐ rén	薏苡仁	10 parts
fù zǐ	附子	2 parts
bài jiàng	敗醬	5 parts

上三味，杵為散，取方寸匕，以水二升，煎減半，頓服，小便當下。

Pestle the three ingredients above into a powder and decoct one gram in 400ml of water until reduced by half. Take in one single dose. Urination should occur immediately.

Song 歌曰:

氣血凝內癰阻外膚，
氣血為內癰所奪，
不榮於外，其身甲錯，
言如鱗甲之交錯也。
腹皮雖急按之濡；
附宜二分苡仁十，
敗醬還須五分驅。

Qì and blood congealed **interior** welling-abscess with obstruction on the skin.
Qì and blood are depleted due to the interior welling-abscess,
and with no nutritive in the exterior, there is encrustation of the body,
so it is said to criss-cross like fish scales.
Although the abdominal skin is soggy when pressed,
two parts *fù zǐ* is appropriate with ten parts *yì yǐ rén*
and five parts *bài jiàng* to drive it out.

Quotation by Wáng Jìnsān 王晉三云:

心氣抑鬱不舒，則氣結於小腸之頭，阻傳道之去路而為癰腫，即《內經》所謂臟不容邪，則還之於腑也。故仲景重用薏苡仁，开通心氣，荣养心境，佐以敗醬，化膿為水；使以附子，一開手太陽小腸之結，一化足太陽膀胱之氣，務令所化之毒，仍從水道而出。精微之奥，豈庸淺者所能推測耶？

[When] heart qì is depressed and constrained, it will be bound in the head of the small intestine, obstructing the circulating path and outlet, resulting in swollen welling-abscesses. Just as the *Huáng Dì Nèi Jīng* says, [when] the viscera are unable to contain evils, they will go into the bowels. Therefore, Zhòngjǐng used a large dose of *yì yǐ rén* to open and free heart qì, and nourish the region of the heart; the assistant *bài jiàng* transforms pus and water; the envoy *fù zǐ* on the one hand opens hand tàiyáng small intestine bind, and on the other transforms foot tàiyáng bladder qì, enforcing the expulsion of transformed toxicity through the waterways. How can it be that [ones with] mediocre and shallow skills are able to speculate on this subtle and profound mystery?

大黃牡丹湯

Dà Huáng Mǔ Dān Tāng

Rhubarb and Moutan Decoction

治腸癰者，少腹腫痞，按之即痛如淋，小便自調，時時發熱，自汗出，復惡寒；其脈遲緊者，膿未成，可下之；脈洪數者，膿已成，不可下之也，此湯主之。

A treatment for intestinal welling-abscess with swelling and glomus in the lesser abdomen, which is painful on pressure, similar to strangury, [with] regular urination, frequent heat effusion, spontaneous sweating, and an aversion to cold. [When there is] a slow and tight pulse, pus has not yet formed, and precipitation can be used. [When there is] a surging and rapid pulse, pus has already formed, and precipitation may not be used. This decoction rules it.[81]

大黃（ 四兩 ）牡丹（ 一兩 ）桃仁（ 五十個 ）冬瓜仁（ 半升 ）芒硝（ 三合 ）

dà huáng	大黃	12g
mǔ dān	牡丹	3g
táo rén	桃仁	50 pcs
dōng guā rén	冬瓜仁	100ml
máng xiāo	芒硝	60ml

上五味，以水六升，煮取一升，去滓，內芒硝，再煎數沸，頓服之。有膿當下，如無膿當下血。

Simmer the five ingredients above in 1,200ml of water until reduced to 200ml. Remove the dregs, add the *máng xiāo*, and simmer again, bringing it to a boil numerous times. Take in one single dose. If pus is present, it will be precipitated, and if there is no pus, blood will be precipitated.

81. This is a slightly condensed version of the original line appearing in the *Jīn Guì Yào Lüè*. The rest of the line goes on to say "....當有血；脈洪數者，脓已成，不可下也。大黃牡丹湯主之。[In this case] there should be blood [in the stool]. With a surging and rapid pulse, pus has already formed, and precipitation may not be used. *Dà Huáng Mǔ Dān Tāng* rules it."

Song 歌曰:

腫居少腹
按之即痛如淋,
小便自調, 時時發熱,
自汗出, 復惡寒。
大腸癰，黄四牡丹一兩從，
冬瓜子仁半升桃五十，
芒硝三合洩腸膿。

[When there is] swelling residing in the lesser abdomen,
immediate pain on pressure similar to strangury,
[but] urination is regulated, [there is] frequent heat effusion,
spontaneous sweating, and an aversion to cold,
[for] large intestine welling-abscess: [use] twelve grams of *dà huáng,* [and] three of *mǔ dān,*
[with] 100ml *dōng guā zǐ rén,* fifty pieces *táo rén,*
and 60ml of *máng xiāo* to drain intestinal pus.

Quotation by Wáng Jìnsān 王晉三云:

肺與大腸相表裏, 大腸癰者, 肺氣下結於大腸之頭, 其道遠於上, 其位近於下, 治在下者因而奪之也。故重用大黄、芒硝開大腸之結, 桃仁、牡丹下將敗之血, 至於清肺潤腸, 不過瓜子一味而已。服之當下血, 下未化膿之血也, 若膿已成形, 肉已壞, 又當先用排膿散及湯。故原文云膿已成, 不可下也。

The lungs and large intestine stand in exterior and interior relationship. [When there are] large intestine welling-abscesses, lung qì has descended and is bound in the head of the large intestine. Its path being far from the upper, but its location being close to the lower [means that] it is treated from below [with precipitation], thereby plundering it. For this reason, large doses of *dà huáng* and *máng xiāo* are used to open the large intestine bind. *Táo rén* and *mǔ dān* descend vanquished blood, in order to clear the lung and moisten the intestines. Now, all that is left is *guā zǐ.* After taking it there should be precipitation of blood. [However, after] precipitation there was no blood [and only] transformation of pus. If pus has already formed, and the flesh has already decayed, then [one] must first take either *Pái Nóng Săn* or *Tāng.* This is the reason why the original line says that if pus has already formed, precipitation may not be used.

王不留行散

Wáng Bù Liú Xíng Sǎn

Vaccaria Powder

治金瘡病。

A treatment for incised wounds.

王不留行（十分，八月八日採）蒴藋細葉（十分，七月七日採）甘草（十八分）桑東南根（白皮十分，三月三日採）黃芩（二分）蜀椒（三分）厚朴（二分）乾薑（二分）芍藥（二分）

wáng bù liú xíng	王不留行	harvested on the 8th day of the 8th month	10 parts
shuò diào xì yè	蒴藋細葉	harvested on the 7th day of the 7th month	10 parts
gān cǎo	甘草		18 parts
sāng dōng nán gēn	桑東南根	[*bái pí*] harvested on the 3rd day of the 3rd month	10 parts
huáng qín	黃芩		2 parts
shǔ jiāo	蜀椒		3 parts
hòu pò	厚朴		2 parts
gān jiāng	乾薑		2 parts
sháo yào	芍藥		2 parts

上九味，王不留行、蒴藋、桑皮三味燒灰存性，各別杵篩，合治之為散，服方寸匕。小瘡即粉之，大瘡但服之。產後亦可服。

Powder the nine ingredients above, and char the *wáng bù liú xíng, shǔ jiāo,* and *sāng pí* to preserve [without destroying] their nature. Pound all the ingredients separately into a powder, and then mix together, taking one gram. For small wounds, apply the powder directly, and for large wounds, take internally. [This] can also be taken by postpartum women.

Song 歌曰:

金瘡諏[82]吉日按春秋而
採不留行，桑蒴同
王不留行按時而取三物，
各十分明，芩樸芍薑均二分，
三分之蜀椒十八分之甘草相成。

[When treating] incised wounds, on an auspicious day in accordance with the seasons,
gather the [*wáng*] *bù liú xíng*, *sāng* [*dōng nán gēn*], and *shuò* [*diào xì yè*] together,
wáng bù liú xíng and the two others are **collected on their respective times**,
ten parts of **each**; two parts each of *huáng qín, hòu pò, sháo yào* and *gān jiāng*;
[and] becoming whole with **three parts of *shǔ jiāo***, and eighteen **parts *gān*** *cǎo*.

Quotation by Yóu Zàijīng 尤在涇云:

金瘡經脈斬絕，營衛阻弛。治之者，必使經脈復行，營衛相貫而後已。

With incised wounds, the channels have been severed, [causing] slack obstruction in the nutritive and defense. One who treats it must restore movement in the channels, [and when there is] passage through the nutritive and defense, [the wound] will resolve.

除燒灰外，餘药不可日曝，火炙方效。

Aside from the charred [medicinals], the remaining medicinals cannot be sun-baked, and are only effective if fire-baked.

Commentary by [Chén] Yuánxī 元犀按:

金刃傷處，封固不密，中於風則瘡口無汁，中於水則出青黄汁，風則發痙，水則濕爛成瘡。王不留行疾行脈絡之血灌溉周身，不使其湍激於傷處，桑根皮洩肌肉之風水；蒴藋葉釋名接骨草，滲筋骨之風水，三者皆燒灰，欲其入血去邪止血也，川椒祛瘡口之風，厚朴燥刀痕之

82. The meaning of *zoū* 諏 here, is "to choose" or "to collect."

濕，黃連退肌熱，芍藥散惡血，乾薑和陽，甘草和陰。用以為君者，欲其入血退腫生肌也。風濕去，陰陽和，瘡口收，肌肉生，此治金瘡之大要。

The area damaged by the incision is not completely sealed. [If the incision is] struck by wind, there will be an absence of fluids [leaking from the sore], and if struck by water, clear yellow fluid will be discharged. With wind there [will be] tetany, and with water, dampness will erode and form sores. ***Wáng bù liú xíng*** quickly moves the blood in the vessels and networks to irrigate the entire body, and prevents the stimulation of rushing fluids to the damaged area. ***Sāng gēn pí*** discharges wind-water from the flesh; ***shuò diào yè***, also called ***jiē gǔ cāo***, percolates wind-water from the sinews and bones. These three medicinals are charred, enabling them to enter the blood, eliminate evils and stop bleeding. ***Chuān jiāo*** dispels wind from the sore opening; ***hòu pò*** dries the dampness in the incision; ***huáng lián*** abates hot flesh; ***sháo yào*** dissipates malign blood; ***gān jiāng*** harmonizes yáng and ***gān cǎo*** harmonizes yīn. When [these medicinals] are used with the sovereign, they are able to enter the blood, reduce swelling, and engender flesh. [When] wind and dampness are eliminated, yīn and yáng will be in harmony, the sore opening will disappear, and flesh will be engendered. These are the main points [to be aware of] when treating incised wounds.

排膿散
Pái Nóng Sǎn
Pus-Expelling Powder

枳實（ 十六枚 ）芍藥（ 六分 ）桔梗（ 二分 ）

zhǐ shí	枳實	16 pcs
sháo yào	芍藥	6 parts
jié gěng	桔梗	2 parts

上三味，杵為散，取雞子黃一枚，以藥散與雞黃相等，揉和令相得，飲和服之，日一服 。

Pestle the three ingredients into a powder and mix equal parts with one egg yolk, and blend evenly. Take with liquid once daily.

Song 歌曰:

排膿散藥本靈臺，
《內經》謂先師
歃血而盟者是。
枳實為君十六枚，
六分芍兮桔二分，
雞黃一個簡而該 。

Pái Nóng Sǎn [was] originally [kept] in the numinous [orchid chamber].[83]
The *Húang Dì Nèi Jīng* says that the teacher of former times[84]
smears his lips with blood when taking an oath [i.e., to swear a sacred oath].[85]
Zhǐ shí is the sovereign at sixteen pieces,

83. The *Líng Tái Lán Shì*《 靈臺蘭室 》(Numinous Orchard Chamber), was where Huáng Dì stored his books.

84. *Xiān shī* 先師 (teacher of former times) could be referring to either Jiù Dàijì 僦貸季, the teacher of an ancestor of Qí Bó, or to an unnamed teacher of Qí Bó or Huáng Dì.

85. This was a method in which teachers of former times would use a blood scribbling ceremony to teach valuable knowledge. *Sù Wèn*, 20: "[I shall] smear blood around my mouth when [I] receive [this knowledge, I will] not dare to let it leak [to others] carelessly". [Unschuld et al.]

with six parts *sháo yào* and two of *jié gěng*,
mixed with one egg yolk; as simple as that!

Commentary by [Chén] Yuánxī 元犀按:

枳、桔行氣滯，芍藥通血滯，從氣血以排之，人所易知也。妙在揉入雞子黃一枚，取有情之物以養心脾之陰，則排之之法，獨得其本也。

Zhǐ shí and *jié gěng* move qì stagnation, while *sháo yào* frees blood stagnation, therefore [pus] is eliminated through the [movement of] blood and qì. This is easy for people to understand. The ingenuity lies in the addition of one egg yolk, as it is an [animal] substance with an affinity to nourish the yīn of the heart and spleen. Only [this] method of [pus] expulsion can capture the root [of the condition].

排膿湯

Pái Nóng Tāng

Pus-Expelling Decoction

甘草（ 二兩 ）桔梗（ 三兩 ）生薑（ 一兩 ）大棗（ 十枚 ）

gān cǎo	甘草	6g
jié gěng	桔梗	9g
shēng jiāng	生薑	3g
dà zǎo	大棗	10 pcs

上四味，以水三升，煮取一升，溫服五合，日再服 。

Simmer the four ingredients above in 600ml of water until reduced to 200ml. Take 100ml warm, two doses per day.

Song 歌曰:

排膿湯與散懸殊，
一兩生薑二草俱，
大棗十枚桔三兩，
通行營衛是良圖 。

There is a major difference between *Pái Nóng Tāng* and *Sǎn.*
Three grams *shēng jiāng* and six grams *gān cǎo* without exception;
ten pieces *dà zǎo,* and nine grams *jié gěng,*
is the right strategy to free and move the nutritive and defense.

Commentary by [Chén] Yuánxī 元犀按:

方中取桔梗、生薑之辛，又取大棗、甘草之甘，辛甘發散為陽，令毒從陽化而出，排之之妙也。

The formula uses acrid *jié gěng,* and *shēng jiāng,* together with sweet *dà zǎo,* and *gān cǎo,* for acrid and sweet [medicinals] are able to effuse and disperse. This is a yáng [method] that causes toxicity to be eliminated through yáng transformation. [This] is an excellent [method] of expulsion.

黃連粉
Huáng Lián Fěn
Coptis Powder

方未見。

Formula has been lost.

治浸淫瘡，從口起流向四肢者可治，從四肢流來入口者不可治 。浸淫瘡，此粉主之 。

In the treatment for wet spreading sores, ones that flow from the mouth to the four extremities are treatable, and those that flow from the four extremities to the mouth are not treatable. For wet spreading sores, this powder rules it.

Song 歌曰:

浸淫瘡藥末黃連，
從口流肢順自然；
若起四肢流入口，
半生常苦毒牽纏 。

[For] wet spreading sores [use] powdered *huáng lián*;
[sores that] flow from the mouth to the four extremities are natural and favorable;
[sores that] flow from the four extremities to the mouth,
would involve a half a lifetime of suffering.[86]

Commentary by [Chén] Yuánxī 元犀按:

浸淫瘡系傳染之疾也。從口起流向四肢者，毒氣外出也，故曰可治。從四肢起流來入口者，毒氣由外入內，固結於臟腑之間，故曰不可治。黃連粉方未見，疑即黃連一味爲末，或敷或服，隨宜擇用。

86. Alluding to the fact that this would be difficult to cure.

Wet spreading sores are an infectious disease. [When they] flow from the mouth to the four extremities, [it] means that toxic qì is about to be expelled and can therefore be treated. [When they] flow from the four extremities to the mouth, it means that toxic qì is entering the interior from the exterior, and is tightly bound within the viscera and bowels, and is therefore not treatable. The formula *Huáng Lián Fěn* has been lost, but it is suspected that powdered *huáng lián* is the only ingredient, and can [either] be applied externally, or ingested, and should be used accordingly.

卷六
Volume Six

趺蹶手指臂腫轉筋陰狐疝蛔蟲方
Fū Jué Shǒu Zhǐ Bì Zhǒng Zhuǎn Jīn Yīn Hú Shàn Huí Chóng Fāng
Formulas for Hobbled Dorsum of the Foot, Swelling in the Fingers and Arms, Cramping, Yīn Fox-like Mounting, and Roundworm Diseases

藜蘆甘草湯
Lí Lú Gān Cǎo Tāng
Veratrum and Licorice Decoction

方未見。

Formula has been lost.

治病人常以手指、臂腫動，此人身體瞤瞤，此湯主之。

A treatment for patients with frequent swelling and stirring of the fingers and arms, and generalized twitching, this decoction rules it.

Song 歌曰:

體瞤臂腫主藜蘆，
癇痹風痰俱可驅；
蘆性升提草甘緩，
症詳方厥遍尋無。

[For] *lí lú* rules body twitching and arm swelling,
[and] expells all seizures, impediment, wind and phlegm;
the nature of *lí lú* is to upbear and rise, while *gān cǎo* moderates with sweetness,
the disease [is] described in detail, [yet] the formula is lost and cannot be found anywhere.

Commentary by [Chén] Yuánxī 男元犀按：

痰涎為濕氣所生，留滯胸膈之間，久則變生無定。云病人常以手指、臂腫動，身體瞤瞤者，是氣被痰阻，濕無去路，或加邪風，風行氣亦行，引動積痰毒氣，此所以群動並發，擾亂心君不甯也。手足項背牽引鈎痛，走易不定者，心君之令不行，肺無以傳其治節也。藜蘆性毒，以毒攻毒，吐久積風痰，殺蟲，通支節，除癇痹也；助用甘草者，取甘潤之意，以其能解百毒也。方雖未見，其意不過是耳。

Phlegm-drool is engendered from damp qì, which stagnates in the space between the chest and diaphragm, and when enduring, will cause a variety of unpredictable changes. [This line] discusses patients with frequent swelling and stirring of the fingers and arms, with generalized twitching, which is due to the obstruction of qì by phlegm. Dampness [phlegm] has no road from which to leave, [and is] occasionally complicated by the addition of wind evil. When wind moves, qì will also move, [which] stirs accumulated phlegm and toxic qì, and [as a result] the various movements [throughout the body] will eventually harrass the heart, leaving the sovereign without peace. This easily leads to pulling tautness and pain of the extremities, neck and back. [When the] sovereign heart is unable to command the lungs they will be unable to convey [their role of] management and regulation. The nature of *lí lú* is toxic [and here] a toxin is used to treat a toxin. [*Lí lú*] is an emetic, used to treat the accumulation of wind-phlegm, kill worms, free the extremities, and eliminate seizures and impediment. This is assisted by the use of *gān cǎo*, where its sweet moistening effect is used to resolve the hundred toxins. Although the formula has never been seen, we can still infer its meaning from the above.

雞屎白散
Jī Shǐ Bái Sǎn
Chicken Feces White Powder

治轉筋病，其人臂腳直，脈上下行，微弦，轉筋入腹者，此散主之。

A treatment for cramping diseases with rigidity of the arms and legs, straight up and down pulses, which are slightly wiry, and [if] cramping enters the abdomen, this powder rules it.

雞屎白為散，取方寸匕，以水六合，和，溫服。

Powder the *jī shǐ bái*, and mix one gram with 120ml of water, and take warm.

Song 歌曰:

轉筋入腹脈微弦，
肝氣凌脾豈偶然？
木畜為雞其屎土，
研來同類妙周旋。

Cramping in the stomach, with a slightly wiry pulse,
is this not [a symptom] of liver qì intimidating the spleen?
The chicken is a wood animal [and] its feces is earth.
Pestle [the feces] to make [it more earth]-like for a wonderful way to contend with this.

Quotation by Yóu Zàijīng 尤在涇云:

《內經》曰：諸暴強直，皆屬於風。轉筋入腹者，脾土虛而肝木乘之也。雞為木畜，其屎反利脾氣，故治是病，且以類相求，則尤易入也。

The *Huáng Dì Nèi Jīng* says that all sudden rigidity is ascribed to wind. Cramping in the stomach is due to a vacuity of spleen earth, [which is] being exploited by liver wood. The chicken is a wood animal, while its excrement disinhibits spleen qì, which is the reason [it is able] to treat this disease. Furthermore, since [chicken feces] belongs to the [earth] class, it can easily enter [the spleen].

蜘蛛散
Zhī Zhū Sǎn
Spider Powder

治陰狐疝氣，偏有小大，時時上下者，主之。

A treatment for yīn fox-like mounting qì,[87] with testicles that change in size, and frequently ascend and descend, [this powder] rules it.

蜘蛛（十四枚，熬焦）桂枝（半兩）

zhī zhū	蜘蛛	boiled until parched	14 pcs
guì zhī	桂枝		1.5g

上二味為散，取八分一匕，飲和服，日再。蜜丸亦可。

Powder the two ingredients above, mix one-eighth of a spoonful of the powder with water, and take twice daily. Mixing the powder with honey to form pills is also acceptable.

Song 歌曰:

陰狐疝氣久難醫，
腎囊為陰病，
則氣之腥臭如狐之臊也。
大小攸偏或偏於左，
或偏於右，一大一小也。
上下時，
時時上下，人多誤解，
謂病發則墜而下，
病息則收而上也。
熬杵蜘蛛十四個，
桂枝半兩恰相宜。

87. The name fox-like mounting is derived from the sly, unpredictable way in which the intestine slides in and out of the scrotum, resembling the way in which a fox slyly slips in and out of its lair. (*A Practical Dictionary of Chinese Medicine*, Wiseman et al. 1998, Paradigm Publications).

Enduring [cases] of yīn fox-like mounting qì are difficult to treat.
Scrotal [issues] are yīn diseases,
and [here] there is a malodorous fish-like smell resembling that of a fox.
There is great variation between the size of the testicles.
Either on the left or the right, one [may be] large, while [the other] small.
[The testicles] ascend and descend frequently.
Frequently ascending and descending, is commonly misunderstood.
The meaning [here] is that [when] the disease emerges there is sagging and descent,
and when the disease is resting, there is contraction and ascent [no sagging].
It is suitable to pestle and simmer fourteen pieces of *zhī zhū*
and one and a half grams *guì zhī* together.

Commentary 按:

此病用桂枝，不如用肉桂力更大。

Guì zhī is used in this disease. However, it would be better to use *ròu guì*, as it is much stronger.

Quotation by Wáng Jìnsān 王晉三云:

蜘蛛性陰而厲，隱見莫測，可定幽暗之風，其功在殼，能洩下焦結氣；肉桂芳香入肝，專散沈陰結疝。《四時刺逆從論》曰：厥陰滑爲狐疝風。推仲景之意，亦謂陰狐疝氣，是陰邪挾肝風而上下無時也。治以蜘蛛，如披郤導窾。

Zhī zhū has a yīn nature which is harsh. It is hidden from view and few can claim a sighting. It can calm gloomy wind, with its power being in the shell, and is able to discharge bound qì in the lower burner. *Ròu guì* is aromatic and enters the liver, [which] specifically dissipates the binding of consolidated yīn [that causes] mounting. *The Discourse on Adverse and Compliant Needling in the Four Seasons,*[88] says [that] when the juéyīn [pulse] is slippery [this is] fox-like mounting wind. In praising [the intention of] Zhòngjǐng's meaning it also says that yīn fox-like mounting qì is [due to] yīn evil, complicated by liver wind with irregularity in ascent and descent. This is treated with *zhī zhū,* [which is] like splitting open a crack and guiding [out evil] through the hole.[89]

88. *Huáng Dì Nèi Jīng Sù Wèn,* Chapter 64.

89. Because *zhī zhū* is an insect, its effect can reach very narrow places in the human body that other medicinals are unable to reach, and thereby assists in the expulsion of evils.

甘草粉蜜湯

Gān Cǎo Fěn Mì Tāng

Licorice, Rice Flour, and Honey Decoction

治蛔蟲病，令人吐涎，心痛發作有時，毒藥不止者，主之。

A treatment for roundworm disease causing drooling and intermittent heart pain; if toxic medicinals have not stopped it, [this decoction] rules it.

甘草（ 二兩 ）白粉（ 一兩 ）白蜜（ 四兩 ）

gān cǎo	甘草	6g
bái fěn	白粉	3g
bái mì	白蜜	12g

上三味，以水三升，先煮甘草，取二升，去滓，內粉蜜攪令和，煎如薄餅，溫服一升，差即止。

For the three ingredients above, use 600ml of water, first simmering the *gān cǎo* until reduced to 400ml. Remove the dregs, add the flour[90] and honey, and mix. Simmer until mixture resembles thin gruel, and take 200ml warm, stopping when cured.

Song 歌曰:

蛔蟲心痛吐涎多，
毒藥頻攻痛不瘥；
一兩白粉二兩甘草四兩蜜，
煮分先後取融和。

Roundworms [have caused] heart pain and copious drooling;
toxic medicinals [have been] frequently [used] to attack, yet the pain fails to reduce.
Three grams of *bái fěn*, six grams of *gān cǎo*, and twelve of honey,
seperately simmered to obtain harmonization.

90. Ground rice or rice flour.

Commentary 按:

鉛粉性善殺蟲，今雜於甘草、白蜜之中，以大甘掩其本性，所謂先誘之而後攻之也。

Qiān fěn[91] is very good at killing worms. In present times it is mixed with *gān cǎo* and honey as their major sweetness can cover up [*qiān fěn's*] inherent [toxic] nature. This is what is referred to as first luring and then attacking.

91. Most scholars believe that the *fěn* 粉 here refers to *bái fěn* (rice flour), however Chén is here referring to *Qiān Fěn* (lead powder), which suggests that it may have been originally used in the formula.

烏梅丸

Wū Méi Wán

Mume Pill

歌解見《傷寒》。

For the song with explanation, see the *Shāng Hán Lùn.*

治蛔厥者，其人當吐蛔，今病者靜而復時煩，此為臟寒，蛔上入膈，故煩，須臾復止；得食而嘔，又煩者，蛔聞食臭出，其人當自吐蛔；蛔厥者，此丸主之。

A treatment for roundworm reversal where there should be vomiting of roundworms. Now the patient is quiet, [but] then [experiences] intermittent vexation. This indicates visceral cold. [When] roundworms ascend into the diaphragm, this results in vexation, which will soon again cease. After eating, there will be retching and vexation once again, as roundworms emerge with the smell of food. Patients [will] spontaneously vomit roundworms; for roundworm reversal, this pill rules.

烏梅（三百個）細辛（六兩）乾薑（十兩）黃連（一斤）當歸（四兩）附子（六兩，炮）川椒（四兩，去汗[92]）桂枝（六兩）人參（六兩）黃柏（六兩）

wū méi	烏梅		300 pcs
xì xīn	細辛		18g
gān jiāng	乾薑		30g
huáng lián	黃連		48g
dāng guī	當歸		12g
fù zǐ	附子	blast-fried	18g
chuān jiāo	川椒	sweated	12g
guì zhī	桂枝		18g
rén shēn	人參		18g
huáng bǎi	黃柏		18g

92. Sweating the medicinal refers to the method of frying the medicinal over a low flame until water and oil begin to effuse outwards.

上十味，異搗篩，合治之，以苦酒漬烏梅一宿，去核，蒸之五升米下，飯熟搗成泥，和藥令相得，內臼中，與蜜杵二千下，丸如梧子大。先食飲服十丸，日三服，稍加至二十丸。禁生冷滑臭等食。

Pound and filter the ten ingredients above separately and combine. Soak the *wū méi* in vinegar overnight, remove the kernels, and steam with 1,000ml of rice. When the rice is cooked, pound to a paste, and blend the medicinals thoroughly and place them in a mortar with honey, and pound them two thousand times. Form into pills the size of firmiana seeds. Take ten pills before meals, three times daily, gradually increasing to twenty pills. Raw cold foods, slimy foods, and malodorous foods are contraindicated.

Quotation by Xú Zhōngkě 徐忠可云:

黄連之苦，可以安蛔，則前甘草與蜜，何以亦能安蛔也？不知上條之蛔，因燥而上逆，致使心痛，故以白粉殺蛔爲主，而加甘、蜜以潤其燥。若蛔厥，未嘗攻心，且蛔因臟寒而上，故以烏梅酸收，黄連苦降，以收伏降蛔爲主，而加辛熱追臟寒。所以一心痛而不吐蛔，一吐蛔而不心痛，此是二條大分別也。

If *huáng lián* is bitter and can calm roundworms, then how is it that the combination of *gān cǎo* and honey as in the previous formula, is also able to calm roundworms? Roundworms in the previous line are the result of dryness and upward counterflow resulting in heart pain, [therefore], *bái fěn* is used to kill the roundworms, and honey and *gān cǎo* are used to moisten dryness. If roundworm reversal has not yet attacked the heart, and moreover the roundworms have ascended due to the visceral cold, the sour and astringing *wū méi* and bitter and descending *huáng lián* are used to subdue and descend the roundworms. With the addition of acrid warm [medicinals], visceral cold is expelled. Therefore, the major difference between these two lines is that one has heart pain and no vomiting of roundworms, and the other has vomiting of roundworms and no heart pain.

婦人妊娠病方
Fù Nü Rèn Shēn Bìng Fāng
Formulas for Diseases in Pregnancy

桂枝湯
Guì Zhī Tāng
Cinnamon Twig Decoction

歌見《傷寒》。

For the song, see the *Shāng Hán Lùn.*

治婦人得平脈，陰脈小弱，其人渴，不能食，無寒熱，名妊娠，此主之。於法六十日，當有此證，設有醫治逆者，卻一月，加吐下，則絕之。

A treatment for women with normal pulses, which are slightly weak in the yīn positions, who are also thirsty, unable to eat, and have an absence of cold or heat; this is called pregnancy, and this [decoction] rules it. As a rule, [these signs] will typically manifest sixty days [following conception]. In the case of [adverse] treatment, vomiting and diarrhea will appear after another month, and this [formula] should be terminated.[93]

Quotation by Xú Zhōngkě 徐忠可云：

桂枝湯表證得之，為解肌和營衛；內證得之，為化氣調陰陽。時醫以薑、桂礙胎戒用，汲汲以養血滋陰為事，皆不知仲景之法也。

Guì Zhī Tāng is used in the contraction of an exterior pattern to resolve the exterior and harmonize the construction and defense. [When] used for the contraction of an interior pattern it transforms qì and regulates yīn and yáng. Current physicians believe that *shēng jiāng* and *guì zhī* may harm

93. Regarding the various commentaries and interpretations of this line, I have opted to translate *jué* 絕 as terminate, referring to the termination of treatment, as opposed to termination of pregnancy, which has been suggested by other commentators.

the fetus, and anxiously concentrate on nourishing the blood and enriching yīn, as they do not understand Zhòngjǐng's methods.

愚按：本章末三句未明，願後之學者補續之。

My own comment: The last three sentences of this line are not clear, and it is my hope that later scholars [will] continue to supplement it.

桂枝茯苓丸

Guì Zhī Fú Líng Wán

Cinnamon Twig and Poria Pill

治婦人宿有癥病，經斷未及三月，而得漏下不止，胎動在臍上者，此為癥痼害。妊娠六月動者，前三月經水利時，胎也。下血者，後斷三月癥也。所以血不止者，其癥不去故也，當下其癥，宜此方主之。

A treatment for women with a history of concretions [that experience] incessant spotting and fetal stirring above the umbilicus within three months after the ceasing of menstruation; this indicates damage from an intractable concretion. If there is fetal stirring in the sixth month of pregnancy, and menstruation was uninhibited in the three months before it ceased, this is the fetus. Descent of blood after an absence [of bleeding] for three months is due to coagulated blood.[94] Therefore, incessant bleeding is caused by the remaining concretion, which should be precipitated, and this pill rules it.

桂枝茯苓丹皮桃仁（去皮尖，熬）芍藥（各等分）

guì zhī	桂枝	use equal parts
fú líng	茯苓	
dān pí	丹皮	
táo rén	桃仁	remove skin, tips, and toast.
sháo yào	芍藥	

上五味末之，煉蜜丸如兔屎大，每日食前服一丸。不知，加至三丸。

Process equal parts of the five ingredients above into a powder and mix with refined honey, forming pills the size of rabbit droppings. Take one pill before meals every day; and if there is no effect, increase to three pills.

94. In the *Jīn Guì Yào Lüè* and various copies of the current text, the character *pēi* 衃 is used, which means coagulated blood. However, in the received text the character *zhèng* 癥 is used, which is translated as concretion. In keeping with Chén's original work I have left the *zhèng* 癥 as is, but have opted to use the translation of coagulated blood.

Song 歌曰:

癥痼未除恐害胎，
胎動於臍下為欲落，
動於臍上是每月湊集之血
因癥痼之氣妨害之而下漏也，
胎安癥去悟新裁；
桂苓丹芍桃同等，
氣血陰陽本末該。

[When] intractable concretions [have] not yet [been] eliminated, [one] fears harming the fetus.
Fetal stirring below the umbilicus means it is about to drop,
stirring above the umbilicus is the gathering and accumulation of blood each month,
which is caused by the qì of [the] intractable concretion resulting in spotting.
In order to calm the fetus and eliminate concretions [one must] comprehend
[that this] composition of equal parts *guì zhī, fú líng, mu dān pí, sháo yào,* and *táo rén,*
[will address] qì, blood, yīn, and yáng, and completely cover the root and tip.

Commentary by Lín Lǐfēng 受業林禮豐按:

師云："婦人宿有癥病"者，謂未受胎之前，本停瘀而有癥病也。"經斷"者，謂經水淨盡之後，交媾而得胎也。"未及三月而得漏下不止"者，謂每月湊集之血因宿昔之癥痼妨害之而下漏也。蓋六月胎動者，胎之常，而三月胎動者，胎之變，然胎當居臍下，今動在臍上者，是本有癥痼在臍下逼動其胎，故胎不安而動於臍上也。因複申言之曰："前三月經水利時，胎也。下血者，後斷三月衃也"。衃者，謂每月湊集之血始凝而未痼也。所以血不止者，其癥不去，必害其胎。去其癥，即所以安其胎，故曰"當下其癥"。主以桂苓丸者，取桂枝通肝陽，芍藥滋肝陰，茯苓補心氣，丹皮運心血，妙在桃仁監督其間，領諸藥抵於癥痼而攻之，使瘀結去而新血無傷。瘀既去，則新血自能養胎，雖不專事於安胎，而正所以安胎也。

The master says "women with a history of concretions," [here] the concretion disease is due to the collection of [blood] stasis prior to conception. "[With] the ceasing of menstruation," sexual intercourse following the elimination of the menstrual flow will result in the conception [of a fetus]. "[In regards to] incessant spotting within three months after the ceasing of menstruation," the spotting is caused by the pre-existing intractable concretion, [which is] impairing the monthly accumulation and gathering of blood. It is normal for there to be fetal stirring in the sixth month of pregnancy, [however] it is abnormal for the fetus to stir in the third month. The fetus should reside below the umbilicus, but now there is stirring above the umbilicus, which means that originally there was an intractable concretion below the umbilicus forcing the fetus to stir. This is the reason for the fetus not being calm and the stirring [to occur] above the umbilicus. This is why it is again emphasized that, "if menstruation was uninhibited in the three months before it ceased, this is the fetus. Descent of blood [after] an absence [of bleeding] for three months is the result of coagulated blood." [Here] the monthly accumulation and gathering of blood is beginning to coagulate and has not yet [formed] an intractable [concretion]. Therefore, because the concretion has not been eliminated there is incessant bleeding, which will invariably harm the fetus. Eliminating the concretion will immediately bring calm to the fetus, which is the reason why it is said that, "[one should] precipitate the concretion." The ruling [formula] ***Guì Zhī Fú Líng Wán*** employs ***guì zhī*** to free liver yáng, ***sháo yào*** to enrich liver yīn, ***fú líng*** to supplement heart qì, ***dān pí*** to move heart blood, and ingeniously maintains it all by adding ***táo rén*** to guide all the medicinals into the concretion [in order] to attack it. This causes the stasis bind to be eliminated, without damage to new blood. Immediately after the stasis is eliminated, new blood will be able to nourish the fetus, resulting in the calming of the fetus. Although [the formula] does not specifically calm the fetus, it can calm it [through this function].

附子湯
Fù Zǐ Tāng
Aconite Decoction

方見《傷寒》。

For the formula, see the *Shāng Hán Lún*.

治婦人懷娠六七月，脈弦發熱，其胎愈脹，腹痛惡寒，少腹如扇，所以然者，子臟開故也，以此湯溫其臟。

A treatment for the sixth or seventh month of pregnancy [with symptoms] of a wiry pulse, heat effusion, increasing distension of the fetus, abdominal pain, aversion to cold, and a feeling in the lesser abdomen as if being fanned, being due to openness of the uterus; this decoction will warm the uterus.

附子（二枚，炮，去皮，破八片）茯苓（三兩）人參（二兩）白朮（四兩）芍藥（三兩）

fù zǐ	附子	blast-fried, skin removed, broken into 8 pcs.	2 pcs
fú líng	茯苓		9g
rén shēn	人參		6g
bái zhú	白朮		12g
sháo yào	芍藥		9g

上五味，以水八升，煮取三升，去滓，溫服一升，日三服。

Simmer the five ingredients above in 1,600ml of water until reduced to 600ml. Remove the dregs and take 200ml warm, three doses per day.

Commentary by [Chén] Yuánxī 男元犀按：

太陽主表，少陰主裏。脈弦發熱者，寒傷太陽之表也。腹痛惡寒者，寒侵少陰之裏也。

Tàiyáng rules the exterior, while shàoyīn rules the interior. A wiry pulse with heat effusion indicates that cold has damaged the exterior [of] tàiyáng. Abdominal pain with an aversion to cold means cold has invaded the interior [of] shàoyīn.

夫胎居臍下，與太少相連，寒侵太少，氣並胞宮，迫動其胎，故胎愈脹也。腹痛惡寒，少腹如扇者，陰邪盛於內，寒氣徹於外，故現出陣陣如扇之狀也。然胎得暖則安，寒則動。寒氣內勝，必致墜胎，故曰所以然者，子臟開故也。附子湯溫其臟，使子臟溫而胎固，自無隕墜之虞矣。附子湯方未見，疑是傷寒附子湯。

The fetus resides below the umbilicus, and is linked by both the tàiyáng and shàoyīn [channels]. [When] cold invades tàiyáng and shàoyīn, the uterus is also impacted, causing stirring of the fetus with even greater distention. When there is abdominal pain and an aversion to cold with a feeling in the lesser abdomen as if fanned, yīn evil is exuberant in the interior and cold qì penetrates the exterior, which is the reason why we see the symptom of rippling which feels as if [one is] being fanned. If the fetus is warm, it will be calm, and will stir if cold. If cold qì prevails in the interior, it will cause a miscarriage, which is the reason why it says that the uterus is open. *Fù Zǐ Tāng* warms the viscera and brings forth warmth to the uterus and secures the fetus, so as to not collapse, thus freeing one from worries! Since the formula has been lost, I suspect it is the [same] *Fù Zǐ Tāng* from the *Shāng Hán Lùn.*

膠艾湯

Jiāo Ài Tāng

Donkey-Hide Gelatin and Mugwort Decoction

治婦人有漏下者，有半產後因續下血都不絕者，有妊娠下血者，假令妊娠腹中痛，為胞阻，以此湯主之。

A treatment for women with [either] spotting, incessant blood descent following late miscarriage, or blood descent in pregnancy. If [there is] abdominal pain in pregnancy, [then] this is uterine obstruction, and this decoction rules it.

乾地黃（六兩）川芎阿膠甘草（各二兩）艾葉當歸（各三兩）芍藥（四兩）

gān dì huáng	乾地黃	18g
chuān xiōng	川芎	6g
ē jiāo	阿膠	6g
gān cǎo	甘草	6g
ài yè	艾葉	9g
dāng guī	當歸	9g
sháo yào	芍藥	12g

上七味，以水五升、清酒三升，合煮取三升，去滓，內膠令消盡，溫服一升，日三服，不差更作。

Simmer the seven ingredients above in 1,000ml of water with 600ml of clear wine, until reduced to 600ml. Remove the dregs, and dissolve the *ē jiāo* in the decoction. Take 200ml warm, three doses per day, and repeat if [the condition] fails to resolve.

Song 歌曰:

妊娠腹滿阻胎胞，
名曰胞阻，以胞中氣血虛寒，
而阻其化育也。
二兩芎藭草與膠，

歸艾各三芍四兩，
地黃六兩去枝梢。

Abdominal fullness in pregnancy with fetal obstruction.
This is called fetal obstruction, which is the result of qì and blood vacuity with cold, which hinders the growth and development of the fetus.
Six grams [each of] *chuān xiōng,*[95] *gān cǎo,* and *ē jiāo,*
nine grams each of *dāng guī* and *ài yè,* twelve of *sháo yào,*
and eighteen of *dì huáng* eliminates the tip of the branch.

Commentary by [Chén] Yuánxī 男元犀按:

芎藭、芍、地，補血之藥也；然血不自生，生於陽明水谷，故以甘草補之。阿膠滋血海，爲胎産百病之要藥；艾葉暖子宮，爲調經安胎之專品，合之爲厥陰、少陰、陽明及衝任兼治之神劑也。後人去甘草、阿膠、艾葉，名爲四物湯，則板實而不靈矣。

Chuān xiōng, sháo yào, and *dì huáng* are blood-supplementing medicinals. Blood is not generated on its own, but is engendered from water and grains in yángmíng; therefore, *gān cǎo* is used to supplement [yángmíng]. *Ē jiāo* enriches the sea of blood, and is a very important medicinal for treating various pregnancy-related diseases. *Ài yè* warms the uterus, and is a specific medicinal to regulate menstruation and calm the fetus. This is a divine formula, which unites juéyīn, shàoyīn, and yángmíng, and simultaneously treats the thoroughfare and controlling vessels. In later times, people have removed the *gān cǎo, ē jiāo* and *ái yé,* renaming it *Sì Wù Tāng,* making this formula stiff, bound, and ineffective!

95. Although the Chinese above says *xiōng qiáng* 芎藭, I have opted to translate this medicinal using its alternate, more common name, *chuān xiōng* 川芎, and it will appear as such in the remainder of the text.

當歸芍藥散
Dāng Guī Sháo Yào Sǎn
Chinese Angelica and Peony Powder

治婦人懷妊，腹中㽲痛，此散主之。

A treatment for dull[96] abdominal pain in pregnant women, this powder rules it.

當歸川芎（各三兩）芍藥（一斤）茯苓白朮（各四兩）澤瀉（半斤）

dāng guī	當歸	9g
chuān xiōng	川芎	9g
sháo yào	芍藥	48g
fú líng	茯苓	12g
bái zhú	白朮	12g
zé xiè	澤瀉	24g

上六味，杵為散，取方寸匕，酒和，日三服。

Grind the six ingredients above into a fine powder, and take one gram with wine, three doses per day.

Song 歌曰:

妊娠㽲痛勢綿綿，
不若寒疝之絞痛、
血氣之刺痛也。
三兩歸芎潤且宣，
芍藥一斤澤減半，
朮苓四兩妙盤旋。

96. The character *jiǎo* 㽲 can be translated two different ways: the first as twisting or sharp [pain], which is how it is translated in various other texts; and the second as dull [pain]. I have opted to translate the character here as dull, as I believe that this is the way that Chén saw it. As can be seen from the accompanying song, he mentions a continuous state of pain, which is neither gripping nor stabbing, suggesting a milder incessant pain. The same character can be seen in the line for *Dāng Guì Shēng Jiāng Yáng Ròu Tāng*, in which the pain is described as incessant.

A state of continuous dull [abdominal] pain in pregnancy,
[this is] neither the gripping pain associated with cold mounting disease,
nor the stabbing pain associated with qì, and blood [stasis]
nine grams each of *dāng guī* and *chuān xiōng* to moisten and furthermore diffuse [blood];
forty-eight grams *sháo yào* and half of *zé xiè,*
[plus] *bái zhú* and *fú líng* at twelve grams apiece wonderfully covers [this].

Commentary by [Chén] Yuánxī 男元犀按：

懷妊腹痛，多屬血虛，而血生於中氣。中者，土也。土過燥不生物，故以歸、芎、芍藥滋之；土過濕亦不生物，故以苓、朮、澤瀉滲之。燥濕得宜，則中氣治而血自生，其痛自止。

Abdominal pain in pregnancy is commonly associated with blood vacuity. Blood is engendered by center qì. The center is earth. When there is excessive dryness of the earth, it is unable to generate anything, so for this reason the enriching medicinals *dāng guī, chuān xiōng,* and *sháo yào* are used. Excess dampness in the earth is also unable to generate anything, so *fú líng, bái zhú,* and *zé xiè* are used to percolate it. When dryness and dampness are appropriately [addressed], center qì will be at peace, blood will be engendered on its own, and pain will cease.

乾薑人參半夏丸
Gān Jiāng Rén Shēn Bàn Xià Wán
Dried Ginger, Ginseng, and Pinellia Pill

治妊娠嘔吐不止，此丸主之。

A treatment for incessant vomiting in pregnancy, this pill rules it.

乾薑人參（各一兩）半夏（二兩）

gān jiāng	乾薑	3g
rén shēn	人參	3g
bàn xià	半夏	6g

上三味末之，以生薑汁糊為丸，桐子大，飲服十丸，日三服。

Process the three ingredients above into a powder and mix with fresh ginger juice, forming into pills the size of firmiana seeds. Take ten pills with water, three doses per day.

Song 歌曰:

嘔吐遷延惡阻名，
妊娠嘔吐，名為惡阻。
胃中寒飲苦相縈；
參薑一兩夏雙兩，
生薑汁糊丸古法精。

Prolonged vomiting is called malign obstruction.
Vomiting in pregnancy is referred to as malign obstruction.
[When] the stomach suffers from the entanglement of cold and rheum,
three grams *rén shēn* and *gān jiāng*, with double of *bàn xià*,
formed into pills with the juice of **fresh** ginger, is the skilled method of the ancients.

Quotation by Yóu Zàijīng 尤在涇云:

陽明之脈，順而下行者也，有寒則逆，有熱亦逆，逆則飲必從之。寒逆用此方，熱逆用外臺方：青竹茹、橘皮、半夏各五兩，生薑、茯苓各四兩，麥冬、人參各三兩，爲治胃熱氣逆嘔吐之法，可補仲師之未備。

The yángmíng vessels normally move downwards. With either cold or heat, they run counterflow, and rheum will typically follow. With counterflow cold use this formula, and with heat counterflow, use the formula from the *Wài Tái*: [which consists of] fifteen grams each of *qīng zhú rú*, *jú pí*, and *bàn xià*; twelve grams each of *shēng jiāng* and *fú líng*, and nine grams [each] of *mài dōng* and *rén shēn*. This [version of the] formula treats qì counterflow vomiting due to stomach heat, which can make up for what was not provided by Master Zhòng[jǐng].

Quotation by Lóu Quánshàn[97] 樓全善云:

余治妊阻病，累用半夏，未嘗動胎，亦有故無隕之義也。

Whenever I treat malign obstruction, I frequently use *bàn xià*, which never stirs the fetus. This is the meaning behind [causing] no harm [to the fetus].[98]

97. A *Míng* Dynasty physician who compiled the *Yī Xué Gāng Mù*《醫學綱目》(The Comprehensive Outline of Medicine). Lóu Quánshàn lived from 1332 to 1401, however, his book was not published until 1565.

98. This passage comes from chapter 71 of the *Huáng Dì Nèi Jīng Sù Wèn*, in which Huáng Dì asks: "When a woman has a double body (is pregnant), how about [treating with] toxic [medicinals]? Qí Bó answers, if there is hardening (concretions), and toxic medicinals are used, [the woman] will not be harmed, and [the fetus] will not be harmed as well."

當歸貝母苦參丸
Dāng Guī Bèi Mǔ Kǔ Shēn Wán
Chinese Angelica, Fritillaria, and Flavescent Sophora Pill

治妊娠小便難，飲食如故者，此丸主之。

A treatment for difficult urination with normal eating and drinking in pregnancy, this pill rules it.

當歸貝母苦參（各四兩）

dāng guī	當歸	12g
bèi mǔ	貝母	12g
kǔ shēn	苦參	12g

上三味末之，煉蜜丸如小豆大，飲服三丸，加至十丸。

Grind the three ingredients above [and mix] with refined honey [to form] pills the size of small beans. Take three pills per dose, increasing [to] up to ten pills [if needed].

Song 歌曰:

飲食如常小便難，
妊娠鬱熱液因乾；
苦參四兩同歸貝，
飲服三丸至十丸。
男子加滑石半兩。

Difficult urination with normal eating and drinking,
[is the result of] depressed heat in pregnancy [which] has dried the fluids.
Kǔ shēn twelve grams, the same of *dāng gūi* and *bèi mǔ*,
take three pills per dose reaching up to ten.
For men, add one and a half grams of *huá shí*.

Commentary by [Chén] Yuánxī 男元犀按:

苦參、當歸補心血而清心火，貝母開肺鬱而瀉肺火。然心火不降，則小便短濇；肺氣不行於膀胱，則水道不通。此方為下病上取之法也。況貝母主淋瀝邪氣，《神農本經》有明文哉。

Both *kǔ shēn* and *dāng guī* supplement heart blood and clear heart fire, while *bèi mǔ* opens lung depression and drains lung fire. If heart fire fails to descend, this will result in short rough voidings of urine; if lung qì fails to move through the bladder, then the waterways will be obstructed. This formula utilizes the method of addressing the upper, to treat lower disease. Moreover, as stated in the *Shén Nóng Běn* [*Cǎo*] *Jīng*, *bèi mǔ* rules the treatment of evil qì strangury with dribbling!

葵子茯苓散
Kuí Zǐ Fú Líng Sǎn
Mallow Seed and Poria Powder

治妊娠有水氣，身重，小便不利，洒淅惡寒，起即頭眩，此散主之。

A treatment for water qì in pregnancy, [with] generalized heaviness, inhibited urination, aversion to cold as after soaking, and dizziness upon rising, this powder rules it.

葵子（一升）茯苓（三兩）

kuí zǐ	葵子	200ml
fú líng	茯苓	9g

上二味，杵為散，飲服方寸匕，日二服，小便利則愈。

Process the two ingredients above by pestling them into a powder. Take one gram per dose, two doses per day. Uninhibited urination means [imminent] recovery.

Song 歌曰:

頭眩惡寒水氣乾，
胎前身重小便難；
均是小便不利，
前責之津乾，
此責之水氣，
水利則濕去身輕矣。
不侵衛陽，則不惡寒矣；
不犯清道，則亦不頭眩矣。
一升葵子苓三兩，
米飲調和病即安。

Dizziness and aversion to cold, water qì assaults.
Prior to delivery [there is] generalized heaviness and difficult urination.

In regards to inhibited urination,
the drying of fluids was the cause in the previous [formula],
and [here] it is caused by water qì.
When water is disinhibited, dampness is eliminated and the body feels light.
Without an invasion [of water qì] on defense yáng, there is no aversion to cold.
Without an invasion [of water qì] on the clear path,[99] there is also no dizziness.
200ml of *kuí zǐ* and nine grams of *fú líng*,
taken mixed with rice, and immediately the disease will be calmed.

Commentary by [Chén] Yuánxī 男元犀按:

葵子俗人畏其滑胎，不必用之。中藏經五皮飲加紫蘇，水煎服，甚效。

When there is fear amongst common people of *kuí zǐ* [causing] habitual miscarriage, it need not be used, and *Wǔ Pí Yǐn*[100] from the *Zhōng Zàng Jīng*[101] can be used with the addition of *zǐ sū*, decocted in water, with excellent results.

99. This is a reference to the head.

100. The original formula was referred to as *Wǔ Pí Sǎn* (Five-Peel Powder).

101. *Zhōng Zàng Jīng* 《中藏經》(Central Treasury Canon from the 2nd century (Eastern *Hàn*)), attributed to Huà Tuó.

當歸散
Dāng Guī Sǎn
Angelica Powder

主治婦人妊娠，宜常服之。

Rules the treatment of pregnant women; [for] it is suitable to regularly take this.

當歸黃芩芍藥川芎（各一斤）白朮（半斤）

dāng guī	當歸	48g
huáng qín	黃芩	48g
sháo yào	芍藥	48g
chuān xiōng	川芎	48g
bái zhú	白朮	24g

上五味，杵為散，酒服方寸匕，日再服；妊娠常服即易產，胎無疾苦；產後百病悉主之。

Process the five ingredients above by pestling them into a powder. Take one gram with liquor, two doses per day. Taken regularly during pregnancy, [this] ensures an easy delivery and a healthy fetus. Also rules the treatment of several postpartum diseases.

Song 歌曰:

妊娠常服之劑，
當以補脾陰為主。
萬物原來自土生，
土中涵濕遂生生；不窮。
一斤芎芍歸滋血，
血爲濕化，胎尤賴之。
八兩朮一斤芩朮本脾藥，
今協血藥而入脾土，
土得濕氣則生物。

又有黃芩之苦寒清肺以主之，
肺氣利則血不滯，
所以生物不息。
大化成。

This is a commonly taken formula in pregnancy,
and rules the supplementation of spleen yīn.
The myriad things are originally engendered from the earth,
and when center earth is moist it fulfills its function of engenderment, **endlessly**.
Forty-eight grams of *chuān xiōng, sháo yào,* and *dāng guī* to enrich the blood,
blood is transformed from moisture, [and the] fetus relies on blood.
[By using] twenty-four grams *bái zhú* and forty-eight of *huáng qín,* ***bái zhú* is a spleen medicinal**
that will assist the blood medicinals in entering spleen earth.
When the earth receives moist qì, then the [myriad] things will be generated.
In addition, *huáng qín* is bitter and cold and rules the clearing of the lungs.
When lung qì moves, then blood will not be stagnant,
allowing for the incessant generation of [the myriad] things;
great transformation will be accomplished.

方義歌中頗詳，不再釋。

The explanation of the formula within the song is quite detailed, so it is superfluous to explain it again.

白朮散

Bái Zhú Sǎn

Atractylodes Macrocephala Powder

主妊娠養胎方。

A ruling formula in pregnancy for nourishing the fetus.

白朮川芎蜀椒（各三分，去汗）牡蠣

bái zhú	白朮		3 parts
chuān xiōng	川芎		3 parts
shǔ jiāo	蜀椒	sweated	3 parts
mǔ lì	牡蠣		no amount given

上四味，杵為散，酒服一錢匕，日三服，夜一服。但苦痛，加芍藥；心下毒痛，倍加芎藭；心煩吐痛不能食飲，加細辛一兩，半夏大者二十枚，服之後，更以醋漿水服之；若嘔，以醋漿水服之複不解者，小麥汁服之；已後渴者，大麥粥服之；病雖愈，服之勿置。

Process the four ingredients above by pestling them into a powder. Take one *qián*-spoons worth with liquor, three doses per day, and one dose at night. With pain, add *sháo yào*; with severe pain below the heart, double the dosage of *chuān xiōng*; with heart vexation, vomiting, pain, and an inability to eat or drink, add three grams of *xì xīn* and twenty large pieces of *bàn xià*. After taking the decoction, drink sour-millet water; if there is retching, drink more sour-millet water, and if it still fails to resolve, take wheat juice. If afterwards there is thirst, eat barley gruel. After the disease resolves, continue taking [barley gruel].

Song 歌曰:

胎由土載朮之功，
養血相資妙有藭，
土以載之，血以養之。
陰氣上凌椒攝下，

白
朮
散

胎忌陰氣上逆，
蜀椒具純陽之性，
陽以陰爲家，
故能攝上焦之熱而下降。
蛎潛龍性得真詮。
牡蛎水氣所結，味鹹性寒，
寒以制熱燎原，
鹹以導龍入海。

Bái zhú strengthens the earth's function of holding the fetus
and is mutually supported by the wonderful *chuān xiōng*, which nourishes the blood.
The [fetus] is held by the earth and nourished by the blood.
Shǔ jiāo absorbs and descends the ascending yīn qì.
The fetus fears the ascending counterflow of yīn qì.
Shǔ jiāo **possesses a pure yáng nature**
and since yáng is rooted in yīn,
it can bring down yáng by absorbing heat in the upper burner.
The true meaning lies [in] *mǔ lì's* subduing dragon nature.
Mǔ lì **[lives in] water qì and has a salty flavor and cold nature.**
Its cold [nature] is able to restrain the heat, which has set the prairie ablaze,[102]
and its salty [flavor] is able to guide the dragon back into the sea.[103]

此方舊本三物各三分，牡蠣闕[104]之。徐靈胎云：原本無分兩。按方下云日三服、夜一服者，牡蠣用一分可也。

In earlier versions of the book, this formula used three parts each of the first three ingredients, while the dosage of *mǔ lì* was missing. Xú Língtāi said that in the original [text], no dosage [for *mǔ lì* was mentioned]. However, according to the formulas method of administration of three doses per day, and one dose at night, using one part *mǔ lì* is acceptable.

102. Insinuating the spreading of heat.

103. Returning fire back to its source.

104. The character *quē* 闕 is the equivalent of the character *quē* 缺, which means deficiency or lack of.

Song for Modifications 加減歌曰：

苦痛芍藥加最美，
心下毒痛倚芎是，
吐痛不食心又煩，
加夏廿枚一細使，
醋漿水須服後吞，
若還不嘔藥可止，
不解者以小麥煮汁嘗，
已後渴者大麥粥喜，
既愈常服勿輕拋，
壺中陰陽大燮理。[105]
按：程雲來云：
以大麥粥調中補脾，
故服之勿置，
非指上藥常服也。
此解亦超。

When one suffers from pain, the addition of *sháo yào* is excellent.
[With] severe pain below the heart, *chūan xiōng* is relied upon;
[with] vomiting, pain, inability to eat, and heart vexation,
twenty pieces of *bán xiá* are meticulously employed,
which should be followed by swallowing sour-millet water.
If the medicinals have still not stopped the vomiting,
and it has not resolved, boil with the juice of wheat.
If there is thirst after it has stopped, [one would] thrive by drinking barley **gruel**.
After the disease resolves, continue taking it [barley gruel] and do not stop,
as this liquid can majorly harmonize central yīn and yáng.
Commentary: Chéng Yúnlái says
that barley gruel can harmonize the center and supplement the spleen,
and should therefore not be cast aside,
which is not referring to the medicinals above.
This explanation is excellent!

方義已詳歌中，不再釋。

The explanation of the formula within the song is quite detailed, so it is superfluous to explain it again.

105. The characters *xiè lǐ* 燮理 carry the meaning of harmonization in regards to treatment.

婦人產後病方

Fù Nü Chǎn Hòu Bìng

Formulas for Postpartum Diseases

小柴胡湯

Xiǎo Chái Hú Tāng

Minor Bupleurum Decoction

歌見《傷寒》。

For the song, see the *Shāng Hán Lùn.*

產婦鬱冒，其脈微弱，嘔不能食，大便反堅，但頭汗出。所以然者，血虛而厥，厥而必冒。冒家欲解，必大汗出，以血虛下厥，孤陽上出，故頭汗出。所以產婦喜汗出者，亡陰血虛，陽氣獨盛，故當汗出，陰陽乃復。大便堅，嘔不能食，小柴胡湯主之。

[When] in postpartum women [there is] veiling depression, a faint and weak pulse, retching, an inability to eat, stools [which are] adversely hard, and sweating only from the head; the reason this is so is because there is a blood vacuity and reversal, and with reversal [there] must be veiling. When veiling patients are about to resolve, there will be great sweating. With blood vacuity there is lower reversal with upward exiting of solitary yáng, manifesting with sweating on the head. Postpartum women have a propensity to sweat, [which leads] to the collapse of yīn and blood vacuity, [with] solitary and exuberant yáng qì. Therefore, only after sweating will yīn and yáng be restored [to balance]. [With] hard stools, vomiting, and an inability to eat, *Xiǎo Chái Hú Tāng* rules it.

Commentary by [Chén] Xīnlán 孫男心蘭按：

產婦脈微弱者，血虛也。血虛而陰不維陽，則為孤陽；陽獨行於上，則頭汗出而冒；陽不及於下，則下厥；陽鬱陰傷，無以養腸胃，故大便堅；陰陽不和，擾動於中，故作嘔而不能食。蓋血虛無以作汗，故鬱冒不得從汗而解也。治之者，當審其病情，以冒家欲解，既不得從頭汗而洩，必得大汗而解者，以小柴胡湯發之，使陽從汗洩，則鬱開而陰陽和矣，此損陽就陰法也。

When a postpartum woman's pulse is faint and weak, this indicates blood vacuity. When the blood is vacuous, yīn is unable to safeguard yáng, which leads to solitary yáng; [when] solitary yáng moves in the upper [body], there is sweating of the head and dizziness; [when] yáng fails to reach the lower, this results in lower reversal; [when] yáng is depressed and yīn is damaged, the intestines and stomach do not receive nourishment, resulting in hard stools; when yīn and yáng are in disharmony, there is a disturbance to the center, which manifests with vomiting and an inability to eat. Here the blood vacuity is unable to cause a sweat, which is the reason why the veiling depression is unable to be resolved through sweating. When treating it, one must assess the situation of the disease. When patients suffer from veiling, if [one] desires to resolve [the disease] which is not draining through the sweat of the head, [one] must obtain a large sweat in order for it to resolve. *Xiǎo Chái Hú Tāng* is used to effuse [sweat] allowing for the [solitary] yáng to be drained through the sweat, [thus] opening the depression and harmonizing both yīn and yáng. This is a method of reducing yáng and moving it towards yīn.

大承氣湯

Dà Chéng Qì Tāng

Major Qì-Coordinating Decoction

見《傷寒論》。

See the *Shāng Hán Lùn.*

治病解能食，七八日更發熱者，此為胃實，宜此湯主之 。

A treatment [for when after] resolution of disease, there is an abilty to eat, but after seven or eight days, heat effusion occurs. This is due to stomach repletion, and this decoction rules it.

當歸生薑羊肉湯

Dāng Guī Shēng Jiāng Yáng Ròu Tāng

Chinese Angelica, Ginger and Mutton Decoction

歌見寒疝。

For the song, see [the section on] "Cold Mounting."

治產後腹中㽲痛者。

A treatment for incessant postpartum abdominal pain.

當歸（三兩）生薑（五兩）羊肉（一斤）

dāng guī	當歸	9g
shēng jiāng	生薑	15g
yáng ròu	羊肉	48g

上三味，以水八升，煮取三升，溫服七合，日三服。若寒多者，加生薑成一斤；痛多而嘔者，加橘皮二兩，白朮一兩。加生薑者，亦加水五升，煮取三升二合，服之。

Simmer the three ingredients above in 1,600ml of water until reduced to 600ml, and take 140ml warm, three doses per day. For patients with an excess of cold, increase the amount of *shēng jiāng* to a total of forty-eight grams. For patients with an excess of pain and retching, add six grams of *jú pí* and three grams of *bái zhú*. If you increase the amount of *shēng jiāng*, also increase the amount of water by 1,000ml, simmer until reduced to 640ml, and take this.

枳實芍藥散

Zhǐ Shí Sháo Yào Sǎn

Unripe Bitter Orange and Peony Powder

主產後腹痛，煩滿，不得臥者 。

Rules [the treatment of] postpartum abdominal pain, vexation, fullness, and sleeplessness.

枳實（ 燒令黑，勿太過 ）芍藥（ 等分 ）

zhǐ shí	枳實	scorched to black, but not excessively	equal parts
sháo yào	芍藥		

上二味，杵為散，服方寸匕，日三服；並主癰膿 。大麥粥下之 。

Process the two ingredients above by pestling equal parts into a powder. Take one gram, three doses per day. Also rules the treatment of welling-abscesses with pus. Take with barley gruel.

Song 歌曰:

滿煩不臥腹疼頻，
枳實微燒芍等平，
羊肉湯方應反看，
彼治虛痛， 此治實痛。
散調大麥粥穩而新 。

Fullness, vexation, sleeplessness, and frequent abdominal pain;
zhǐ shí slightly charred with equal parts *sháo yào,*
should be seen as the opposite of the formula *Yáng Roù Tāng,*
which treats vacuity pain, while this formula treats repletion pain.
It is safe and creative to use the powder mixed with barley **gruel**.

Commentary by [Chén] Wèi 男蔚按:

枳實通氣滯，芍藥通血滯，通則不痛，人所共知也。妙在枳實燒黑，得火化而善攻停積；下以大麥粥，和肝氣而兼養心脾，是行滯中而寓補養之意，故癰膿亦主之。

Zhǐ shí frees qì stagnation, while *sháo yào* frees blood stagnation. Free flow results in the absence of pain, which is common knowledge amongst the people. The ingenuity [of this formula] lies in the charring of *zhǐ shí,* which when transformed by fire, becomes excellent at attacking collections and accumulations. [When] taken with barley gruel, liver qì is harmonized, while the heart and spleen are simultaneously nourished. The intention [of this formula] is to move stagnation while supplementing and nourishing, which is the reason it also rules the treatment of welling abscesses with pus.

下瘀血湯

Xià Yū Xuè Tāng

Stasis Purging Decoction

治產婦腹痛，法當以枳實芍藥散，假令不愈者，此為腹中有瘀血著臍下，宜此湯，亦主經水不利 。

When treating postpartum abdominal pain, as a rule, *Zhǐ Shí Sháo Yào Sǎn* is given, but if it fails to resolve [it], then it is due to static blood in the abdomen below the umbilicus and this decoction is suitable. It also rules the treatment of inhibited menstruation.

大黃（ 三兩 ）桃仁（ 二十個 ）蟅蟲（ 二十枚，去足，熬 ）

dà huáng	大黃		9g
táo rén	桃仁		20 pcs
zhè chóng	蟅蟲	remove the legs and boil	20 pcs

上三味末之，煉蜜和為四丸，**以酒一升煮一丸，**取八合，頓服之 。新血下如豚肝 。**各本略異。**

Process the three ingredients above into a powder and combine with refined honey to form four pills. **Simmer one pill in 200ml of liquor** until reduced to 160ml, and take it by drinking it down in one gulp. The color of the freshly precipitated blood should resemble the color of pig liver. **There are slight variances in other versions of the text.**

Song 歌曰:

臍中著痛瘀為殃，
廿粒桃仁三兩黃，
更有蟅蟲二十個，
酒煎大下亦何傷？

[In this type] of umbilical pain, stasis is taken to be the calamity.
Twenty pieces of *táo rén* and nine grams *dà huáng*,

furthermore with twenty pieces of *zhè chóng*,
for when [these medicinals] are brewed in liquor, how could great precipitation be damaging?

Commentary by [Chén] Yuánxī 男元犀按:

服枳實、芍藥而不愈者，非積停不通，是瘀結不散，用此方攻之。方中大黄、桃仁能推陳下瘀；蟅蟲之善攻乾血，人盡知之；妙在桃仁一味，平平中大有功力。鬱血已敗而成瘀，非得生氣不能流通。桃得三月春和之氣，而花最鮮明似血，而其生氣皆在於仁，而味苦又能開洩，故宜人血中而和之散之，逐其舊而不傷其新也。

If there is no recovery after taking *zhǐ shí* and *sháo yào,* [it is] not due to obstruction and collection of accumulations, but [is the result] of static bind [which] has not been dissipated, and this formula is used to attack it. In the formula, *dà huáng* and *táo rén* are able to push out the old [by] precipitating stasis, while it is known that *zhè chóng* is very good at attacking dry blood. The ingenuity lies in *táo rén,* which while being an ordinary [medicinal] can exert profound results. Depressed blood has already decayed and [has now] become static, and without vital qì, it is unable to flow freely. *Táo rén* accepts the harmonious spring qì of the third month, and its flower distinctly resembles [the color of] blood. [At this time] its energy is collected in the seeds, and with its bitter flavor, it is able to open and discharge. This is the reason why [*táo rén*] is able to [enter] the blood [aspect] and both harmonize and dissipate, by expelling the old, and not allowing damage to the new.

大承氣湯

Dà Chéng Qì Tāng

Major Qì-Coordinating Decoction

治產後七八日，無太陽症，少腹堅痛，此惡露不盡；不大便，煩躁發熱，切脈微實，再倍發熱，日晡時煩躁者，不食，食則譫語，至夜即愈，宜此湯主之。熱在裏，結在膀胱也。

A treatment for women who seven or eight days after giving birth have no táiyáng signs, [but have] hard pain in the lesser abdomen, this indicates incomplete elimination of lochia. If there is constipation, vexation, agitation, heat effusion, slightly replete pulses, aggravated heat effusion, and vexation and agitation in the late afternoon, there will be an inability to eat or delirious speech after eating. The condition will resolve by the evening. This decoction rules it, as there is heat in the interior, and binding in the bladder.

Commentary by [Chén] Xīndiǎn 孫男心典按：

無太陽症者，外無病也。脈微實、煩躁發熱、食則譫語者，胃熱也。惡露不盡者，主太陽之氣隨經也。蓋膀胱接胃，連於少腹，血結其所，熱聚其中，宜此湯以下瘀除熱。

In the absence of any tàiyáng signs, the exterior is not diseased. [When] the pulse is slightly replete, with vexation, agitation, heat effusion, and delirious speech following eating this is [due to] stomach heat. Incomplete elimination of lochia is ruled by the qì of tàiyáng, which [should flow] from its channel. Now, the bladder and stomach are connected in the lesser abdomen, which is where the blood is bound, and heat has accumulated, and this decoction is suitable to precipitate stasis and eliminate heat.

陽旦湯
Yáng Dàn Tāng
Yáng Dawn Decoction

治產後中風續續數十日不解，頭微疼，惡寒，時時有熱，心下悶，乾嘔汗出，雖久陽旦症續在者，可與之。

A treatment for postpartum wind strike that remains unresolved for several tens of days, with a mild headache, aversion to cold, frequent heat effusion, oppression below the heart, dry retching, and sweating. Even though [the condition] has persisted for a long time, *Yáng Dàn Tāng* signs are still present, and can thus be given. [This formula] is *Guì Zhī Tāng* with increased *guì zhī* and the addition of *fù zǐ*.

即桂枝湯增桂加附。坊本謂加黄芩者，未知《傷寒論》太陽篇中已明其方，孫真人及各家俱誤。桂枝湯見《傷寒論》。

In old block-printed versions of the text[106] this formula was thought to be [*Guì Zhī Tāng*] with the addition of *huáng qín*, as these texts were unclear whether this was the same formula mentioned in the tàiyáng chapter of the *Shāng Hán Lùn*. Master Sūn Sīmiǎo and [various] others have made this mistake. For *Guì Zhī Tāng*, see the *Shāng Hán Lùn*.

Commentary by [Chén] Yuánxī 男元犀按：

頭痛發熱、惡寒汗出，太陽表症也。心下悶者，太陽水邪彌漫心下而作悶也。陽旦湯即桂枝湯倍桂枝加附子。雖產後數十日不解，其邪仍在於太陽之經，故仍用桂枝湯解太陽之表邪，加桂以化膀胱之水氣，加附子以溫固水臟，使經臟氣化，則內外之邪出矣。

Headache, heat effusion, aversion to cold, and sweating are symptoms associated with a tàiyáng exterior pattern. [With] oppression below the heart, tàiyáng water evil pervades [the area] below the heart and causes oppression. *Yáng Dàn Tāng* is *Guì Zhī Tāng* with double the *guì zhī* and the addition of *fù zǐ*. Although there is a lack of resolution ten days postpartum, evils are still located

106. The old 'block printed' versions of the text are most likely a reference to the *Qiān Jīn Yào Fāng*《千金要方》and the various works of Yù Jiāyán 喻嘉言. They were referred to as block printed versions, as they were not considered to be official copies of the *Shāng Hán Lùn* or the *Jīn Guì Yào Lüè*.

in the tàiyáng channel, and it is for this reason that *Guì Zhī Tāng* is used to resolve exterior evil in the tàiyáng. *Guì zhī* is increased in order to transform water qì in the bladder. *Fù zǐ* is added to the formula to warm and secure the water viscus, enabling the transformation of qì in the channels and viscera, and ensuring the expulsion of evils in both the interior and exterior.

《傷寒論》桂枝加附子，治漏汗；加桂，治氣從少腹上衝心；去芍，治胸滿，俱有明文可據。孫真人以桂枝湯加黃芩爲陽旦湯，其意以心下悶爲熱氣，誤矣。夫有熱氣，則當心煩，今日心下悶，則非熱可知矣。況微惡寒時時有熱，乾嘔汗出，爲太陽桂枝湯之的症。蓋太陽底面便是少陰，續續至數十日不解，顯系少陰之君火微，而水寒之氣盛，寒氣上淩陽位，是以爲心下悶之苦。故取桂枝湯增桂以扶君主之陽，加附子以鎮水陰之逆，使心陽振，水臟溫，則上逆之陰邪，不攻而自散矣。

In the *Shāng Hán Lùn*, *Guì Zhī Jiā Fù Zǐ Tāng* is used to treat leaking sweat; increasing *guì zhī* treats surging qì from the lesser abdomen into the heart, and removing *sháo yào* treats chest fullness. These [principles] are in accordance with the [original] writings. [According to] Master Sūn [Sīmiǎo], *Yáng Dān Tāng* is *Guì Zhī Jiā Huáng Qín Tāng*, [as he felt that] oppression below the heart was due to hot qì; this is a mistake! Now if there were hot qì, then there would be heart vexation, [but] presently with the oppression below the heart, we know there is no heat! Moreover, slight aversion to cold, and frequent heat [effusion], dry retching, and sweating, is a *Guì Zhī Tāng* tàiyáng presentation. In all [cases] of tàiyáng, there is shàoyīn at the bottom, and with continuous [wind strike] reaching ten days without resolution, there is a clear relation to the debilitation of shàoyīn sovereign fire, with exuberance of cold water qì. Cold qì ascends and encroaches into the position of yáng, resulting in oppression below the heart. Therefore, *Guì Zhī Tāng* with increased *guì zhī* supports sovereign yáng, and with the addition of *fù zǐ*, counterflow of water yīn is settled, heart yáng is vitalized, and the water viscus is warmed. Then, ascending counterflow of yīn evil will not attack, and dissipates on its own!

竹葉湯

Zhú Yè Tāng

Bamboo Leaf Decoction

治產後中風，發熱，面正赤，喘而頭痛者，此湯主之。

A treatment for postpartum wind strike, heat effusion, a full red facial complexion, panting, and headaches, this decoction rules it.

竹葉（一把）葛根（三兩）防風桔梗桂枝人參甘草（各一兩）附子（一枚，炮）生薑（五兩）大棗（十五枚）

zhú yè	竹葉		one handful
gé gēn	葛根		9g
fáng fēng	防風		3g
jié gěng	桔梗		3g
guì zhī	桂枝		3g
rén shēn	人參		3g
gān cǎo	甘草		3g
fù zǐ	附子	blast-fried	1 pc
shēng jiāng	生薑		15g
dà zǎo	大棗		15 pcs

上十味，以水一斗，煮取二升半，分溫三服，溫覆使汗出。

Simmer the ten ingredients above in 2,000ml of water, until reduced to 500ml. Divide and take warm in three doses. Cover up to keep warm and promote sweating.

頸項強，用大附子一枚，破之如豆大，前藥揚去沫。嘔者，加半夏半升洗。

[When there is] rigidity of the neck and nape, use one large piece of *fù zǐ*, broken into bean sized pieces. [Simmer] before the [other] ingredients, and remove the foam collecting on top. [If there is] retching, add 100ml of washed *bàn xià*.

Song 歌曰:

喘熱頭疼面正紅，勢欲成痙。
一兩防桔桂草參同，同用一兩。
葛根三兩生薑五兩附枚一，
棗十五枚竹葉一把充 。

Panting, heat, headache, and full red facial complexion, **with a tendency to turn into spasms,**
[use] **three [grams]** *fáng fēng, jié gěng, guì zhī, gān cǎo,* and *rén shēn* **alike three grams of each.**
Nine grams of *gé* ***gēn***, fifteen of ***shēng*** *jiāng,* and one piece of *fù zǐ,*
with fifteen pieces of *dà zǎo* and a handful of *zhú* ***yè***!

Song for Modifications 加減歌曰:

頸項強用大附抵，
以大易小不同體；
嘔為氣逆更議加，
半夏半升七次洗 。

[When there is] rigidity of the neck and nape, use a large piece of pounded *fù zǐ;*
a larger [piece is used] as opposed to a smaller [one], as [this is] a different pattern.
[When there is] retching due to qì counterflow, further modification is suggested;
[use] 100ml of *bàn xià* washed seven times.

Quotation by Chéng Yúnlái 程雲來云:

證中未至背反張，而發熱面赤頭痛，亦風痙之漸。故用竹葉主風痙，防風治內痙，葛根療剛痙，桂枝治柔痙，生薑散風邪，桔梗除風痹，辛以散之之劑也；又佐人參生液以養筋，附子補火以致水，合之甘草，以和諸藥，大棗以助十二經。同諸風劑，則發中有補，為產後中風之大劑也。

A condition that has not yet [become] as severe as arched-back rigidity, but that has heat effusion, a red facial complexion, and headaches, is the beginning of wind tetany. Therefore, *zhú yè* is used [as it] rules wind tetany, *fáng fēng* treats internal tetany, *gé gēn* treats hard tetany, and *guì zhī* treats soft tetany. *Shēng jiāng* dissipates wind evil, while *jié gěng* eliminates wind impediment. This prescription utilizes acrid [medicinals] in order to dissipate. In addition, these are assisted by *rén shēn,* which engenders fluids to nourish the sinews, and *fù zǐ,* which supplements fire in order to produce water. These [are all] combined with *gān cǎo,* which harmonizes all the medicinals, and *dà zǎo,* which assists all twelve channels. All together [this is a] wind prescription, which [contains ingredients] to effuse and [at the same time] supplement, making it a major prescription for postpartum wind strike.

竹皮大丸
Zhú Pí Dà Wán
Major Bamboo Shavings Pill

治婦人乳中虛，煩亂嘔逆，安中益氣。

A treatment for vacuity in women during lactation, with vexing confusion and retching counterflow; [this formula will] calm the center and boost qì.

生竹茹石膏（各二分）桂枝白薇（各一分）甘草（七分）

zhú rú	竹茹	2 parts
shí gāo	石膏	2 parts
guì zhī	桂枝	1 part
bái wēi	白薇	1 part
gān cǎo	甘草	7 parts

上五味末之，棗肉和丸彈子大，飲服一丸，日三夜二服。有熱，倍白薇；煩喘者，加柏實一分。

Process the five ingredients above into a powder, and combine with *dà zǎo,* forming into bullet-sized pills. Take one pill with water, three doses per day and two at night. With heat, double the dosage of *bái wēi.* With vexation and panting, add one part *bǎi shí.*[107]

Song 歌曰：

嘔而煩亂乳中虛，
謂乳子之時，氣虛火勝，
內亂而上逆也。
二分石膏與竹茹，
薇桂一分兮草七分，
棗丸飲服效徐徐。

107. *Bái shǐ* (Semen Platycladi).

Vacuity during lactation with retching and vexing confusion.
It is said that at the time of lactation, qì is vacuous and fire is exuberant, resulting in internal confusion and ascending counterflow.
Two parts *shí gāo* and *zhú rú*;
one **part** *bái wēi* and *guì zhī*, yes, and seven parts *gān cǎo*,
for when taken as a pill made with the meat of *dà zǎo*, the effects will be gradual.

Song for Modifications 加減歌曰：

白薇退熱絕神異，
有熱倍加君須記；
柏得金氣厚且深，
葉葉西向歸本位，
實中之仁又寧心，
煩喘可加一分餌。

Bái wēi's [ability to] abate heat is superb and magical,
[so] it must be remembered that [*bái wēi*] should be doubled in the presence of heat!
Bǎi shí can capture the thick and yet sinking metal qì
[for its] leaves face towards the west, [thus] returning to the [metal qì's] root position.
The kernel [of *bǎi*] *shí* also tranquilizes the heart,
[so with] vexation and panting, one part should be added.

Commentary by [Chén] Yuánxī 男元犀按：

血者，中之所生也；乳者，血之所變也。血雖生於中焦，尤藉厥少之氣傳變而為乳。乳中虛者，謂乳子去汁過多而致虛也。中虛無血奉心則煩，心神不安則亂，陽氣上升則嘔。逆者，嘔之甚也。用竹皮大丸者，以竹茹降逆止嘔，白薇除熱退煩，石膏通乳定亂，重用甘草、大棗定安中焦以生津液，血無陽氣不運，妙以桂枝一味，運氣血奉心通乳，則嘔逆止而中即自安，煩亂退而氣即自益矣。復申明其立方之本意曰安中益氣。竹皮大丸，神哉！

Blood is engendered in the center; breast milk is transformed from blood. Although blood is engendered in the middle burner, it is by the means of the qì of juéyīn that it is transmitted and transformed into breast milk. [When there is] vacuity in lactation, it is said that the excessive suckling of milk by the child will result in vacuity. [When] the center is vacuous, blood is unable to nourish the heart resulting in vexation, and when there is disquietude of the heart spirit, there will be confusion. When yáng qì ascends, this will result in retching. When there is counterflow, the retching will be severe. [For this] ***Zhú Pí Dà Wán*** is used, as ***zhú rú*** is able to downbear counterflow and stop vomiting; ***bái wēi*** eliminates heat and abates vexation; ***shí gāo*** frees milk and settles confusion, and a large dose of ***gān cǎo*** is used with ***dà zǎo*** to stabilize and calm the middle burner in order to engender fluids. Blood is unable to move without yáng qì, which is why ***guì zhī*** is ingeniously added to move qì and blood, revere the heart, and free the milk. As a result, the retching counterflow will stop, the center will immediately be calmed on its own, vexing confusion will be abated, and qì will be boosted naturally. Again, to declare the core meaning of the formula, [Zhòngjǐng] proclaimed that it calms the center and boosts qì. ***Zhú Pí Dà Wán*** is like magic!

白頭翁加甘草阿膠湯

Bái Tóu Wēng Jiā Gān Cǎo Ē Jiāo Tang

Pulsatilla Decoction plus Licorice and Gelatin

治產後下利虛極者，此湯主之。

A treatment for postpartum diarrhea and extreme vacuity, this decoction rules it.

白頭翁阿膠甘草（各二兩）黃連黃柏秦皮（各三兩）

bái tóu wēng	白頭翁	6g
ē jiāo	阿膠	6g
gān cǎo	甘草	6g
huáng lián	黃連	9g
huáng bǎi	黃柏	9g
qín pí	秦皮	9g

上五味，以水七升，煮取三升，去滓，入阿膠，更上微火煎膠烊消，取二升，溫服一升，不愈，更服一升。

Simmer the five ingredients above in 1,400ml of water until reduced to 600ml. Remove the dregs, add the *ē jiāo,* and again place on low heat, melting the *ē jiāo* and reducing the water to 400ml. Take 200ml warm, and if [the condition] does not resolve, take another 200ml.

Song 歌曰:

白頭方見傷寒歌，
二兩阿膠甘草和，
產後利成虛已極，
滋阿膠救其陰。
而且緩甘草緩其急。莫輕過。

For the *bái tóu* [*wēng*] formula, see the *Shāng Hán* song;[108]
add six grams each of *ē jiāo* and *gān cǎo*;
for postpartum diarrhea resulting in extreme vacuity;
enrich **[with]** ***ē jiāo*** **[to] rescue the yīn**,
as well as moderate, [for] ***gān cǎo*** **moderates urgency,** do not overlook [its effectiveness].

Commentary by [Chén] Yuánxī 男元犀按:

產後去血過多，又兼下利亡其津液，其為陰虛無疑，兹云虛極，理宜大補，然歸、芎、芍、地則益其滑而下脫，參、朮、桂、芪則動其陽而上逆，皆爲禁劑。須知此“虛”字，指陰虛而言，與少陰證陰氣欲絕同義。少陰證與大承氣湯急下以救陰，與此證與白頭翁大苦以救陰同義。此法非薛立齋、張景嶽、李士材輩，以甘溫爲主、苦寒爲戒者所可窺測。尤妙在加甘草之甘，合四味之苦，爲苦甘化陰法；且久利膏脂盡脫，脈絡空虛，得阿膠之滋潤，合四味之苦以堅之，則源流俱清，而利自止。

With postpartum excessive blood loss and simultaneous diarrhea, [there will be] collapse of fluids and undoubtedly yīn vacuity. This is referred to as extreme vacuity, which should be rectified with major supplementation, and if [medicinals such as] *dāng guī, chuān xiōng, sháo yào,* and *dì huáng* [are used] they can increase the efflux and cause downward desertion. [If] *rén shēn, bái zhú, guì zhī,* and *huáng qí* [are used], they can stir yáng [and cause] ascending counterflow. These are all prohibited. It must be known that the character *xū* 虛 (vacuity) here refers to yīn vacuity, which has the same meaning as a shàoyīn pattern, with yīn qì on the verge of expiry. Precipitating urgently with *Dà Chéng Qì Tāng* in a shàoyīn pattern to rescue yīn, has the same meaning as administering the majorly bitter *bái tóu wēng* in this pattern in order to rescue yīn. This is not a method that people like Xuē Lìzhāi, Zhāng Jǐngyuè, or Lǐ Shìcái could understand, as they [would] use sweet and warm [medicinals] as their ruling principle and were afraid of using bitter and cold [medicinals]. It is a particularly ingenious method to combine sweet *gān cǎo* with the four bitter medicinals in order to form yīn [using] bitter and sweet [medicinals]. Moreover, enduring diarrhea [will result in] extreme desertion of one's riches,[109] and thereby [leave the] vessels and networks empty and vacuous. Give the enriching and moistening *ē jiāo* in combination with the four bitter and hardening medicinals and [both] the source and development [of the condition] will be cleared and the diarrhea will stop on its own.

---

108. This is most likely a reference to the *Cháng Shā Fāng Gē Kuò*《長沙方歌括》(Formulas with songs from Cháng Shā), a companion book of commentaries and songs on the *Shāng Hán Lùn* formulas written by Chén Xiūyuán.

109. One's yīn.

附方
Fù Fāng
Attached Formulas

《千金》三物三黃湯
Qiān Jīn Sān Wù Sān Huáng Tāng
Three Ingredients Three Yellows Decoction from the *Qiān Jīn Yào Fāng*[110]

治婦人在草蓐，自發露得風，四肢苦煩熱，頭痛者，與小柴胡湯；頭不痛但煩者，此湯主之。

A treatment for women suffering from vexing heat in the extremities after contracting wind while on a straw childbed. If there is headache, give *Xiǎo Chái Hú Tāng*. If there are no headaches and only vexation, this decoction rules it.

黃芩（一兩）苦參（二兩）乾地黃（四兩）

huáng qín	黃芩	3g
kŭ shēn	苦參	6g
gān dì huáng	乾地黃	12g

上三味，以水六升，煮取二升，溫服一升，多吐下蟲。

Simmer the three ingredients above in 1,200ml of water until reduced to 400ml, and take 200ml warm. [This formula may cause] profuse vomiting or precipitation of worms.

Song 歌曰:

婦人發露得風傷，
頭不痛兮證可詳，

110. This same formula is referred to as *Qiān Jīn Sān Wù Huáng Qín Tāng*《千金》三物三黃湯 in the *Jīn Guì Yào Lüè*.

肢苦但煩芩一兩，
地黃四兩二苦參良。

[When] women [suffer] damage [following] exposure and contraction of wind,
yet the head is not painful, other patterns [must be] carefully [examined; when]
only suffering from vexation in the extremities, three grams *huáng qín*,
twelve of *dì huáng*, and six of ***kǔ** shēn* will suffice!

Commentary by Lín Lǐfēng 受業林禮豐按:

《千金》云：婦人在草蓐，是新產時也。新產血虛，厥陰主血，血虛則厥陰之相火動，火動則毛竅開。因自發去衣被，露其身體，風邪遂乘虛而襲焉。夫風爲陽邪，四肢爲諸陽之本，兩陽相搏，故四肢苦煩熱也。頭痛者，風邪從臟而乾於腑，有欲外出之象，故與小柴胡湯達之，使其從樞以外出也。頭不痛但煩者，風邪內鬱，擾動心包之熱，心包火熾，血液必傷，故主以三黃湯。取地黃之甘寒多液者，補陰血之虛；黃芩、苦參之苦寒者，瀉心包之熱，使火平而風熄，陰複則肝寧，何有四肢苦煩熱之病哉？且心包有熱，必挾風木而生蟲，故方下云：服後多吐下蟲。

The *Qiān Jīn Fāng* says that when women have just given birth, they lie on straw childbeds, and at this time, their blood is vacuous. Juéyīn rules the blood. When blood is vacuous, juéyīn ministerial fire will stir, and when [this] fire stirs, the pores will be open. [If one] spontaneously removes their clothing and blankets, the body will be exposed, and wind evil will subsequently exploit the vacuity and attack. Now, wind is a yáng evil, and the four extremities are the root of all yáng. When there is struggle between these two yángs [this will] result in vexing heat of the four extremities. When there is headache, wind evil [travels] from the viscera and assaults the bowels, and this should be expelled outwards. Therefore, *Xiǎo Chái Hú Tāng* is given to outthrust evil, which will allow it to be expelled outward from the pivot. If there are no headaches, and only vexation, wind evil is depressed internally and agitates the heat within the pericardium. When pericardium heat is intense, blood will be damaged, and therefore *Sān Huáng Tāng* is the ruling [formula]. *Dì huáng* is used for it is sweet and cold with abundant thick fluids, which supplements vacuity of both yīn and blood; *huáng qín* is bitter and cold, which can drain heat in the pericardium, allowing for the pacifying of fire and extinguishing of wind. When yīn is restored, the liver will be peaceful, and then how could there be vexing heat in the four extremities? Moreover, [when] there is heat in the pericardium this will be complicated by wind-wood, which will engender worms. This is the reason why below the formula the text says that after taking, it may cause profuse vomiting or precipitation of worms.

《千金》內補當歸建中湯

Qiān Jīn Nèi Bǔ Dāng Guī Jiàn Zhōng Tāng

Chinese Angelica Interior Supplementing
Center-Fortifying Decoction from the *Qiān Jīn Yào Fāng*

治產後虛羸不足，腹中刺痛不止，吸吸少氣，或苦少腹急攣痛引腰背，不能飲食；產後一月，日得服四五劑為善，令人強壯宜。

A treatment for postpartum vacuity emaciation and insufficiency with incessant stabbing pain in the center of the abdomen, shortage of qì in spite of heavy inhalations, possibly with hypertonicity and pain in the lesser abdomen stretching to the lower back and back, and an inability to eat or drink. Over the first month following delivery, it is a good idea to take four or five doses throughout the day, as it will provide [the woman] with strength.

當歸（四兩）桂枝（三兩）芍藥（六兩）生薑（三兩）甘草（二兩）大棗（十二枚）

dāng guī	當歸	12g
guì zhī	桂枝	9g
sháo yào	芍藥	18g
shēng jiāng	生薑	9g
gān cǎo	甘草	6g
dà zǎo	大棗	12 pcs

上六味，以水一斗，煮取三升，分溫三服，一日令盡。若大虛，加飴糖六兩，湯成納之，於火上暖令飴消。若去血過多，崩傷內衄不止，加地黃六兩，阿膠二兩，合八味，湯成納阿膠。若無當歸，以芎藭代之。若無生薑，以乾薑代之。

Simmer the six ingredients above in 2,000ml of water until reduced to 600ml, divide, and take three doses warm per day. If there is major vacuity, add eighteen grams of *yí táng* to the decoction and bring back under a low flame until dissolved. With excessive blood loss, flooding, or incessant spontaneous internal bleeding, add eighteen grams of *dì huáng* and six grams of *ē jiāo*. Combine the ingredients and add the *ē jiāo* once the decoction is complete. If there is no *dāng guī*, replace with *chuān xiōng*. If there is no *shēng jiāng*, replace with *gān jiāng*.

Song 歌曰:

補中方用建中湯，
四兩當歸去瘀良；
產後虛羸諸不足，
調榮止痛補勞傷。

To supplement the center, a useful formula is *Jiàn Zhōng Tāng*;
[adding] twelve grams *dāng guī* is excellent for removing stasis.
[In] postpartum vacuity, marked emaciation, and the various insufficiencies,
[it] regulates the nutritive, stops pain, and supplements taxation damage.

Song for Modifications 加減歌曰:

服湯行瘀變崩傷，
二兩阿膠六地黃；
若厥生薑宜變換，
溫中止血宜乾薑；
當歸未有川芎代，
此法微茫請細詳。

Take this decoction to move stasis. If [now there is] flooding,
[add] six grams of *ē jiāo* and eighteen of *dì huáng*.
If there is reversal, it is suitable to replace the *shēng jiāng*,
[in order to] warm the center and stop bleeding it is suitable [to use] *gān jiāng*.
In the absence of *dāng guī*, replace with *chuān xiōng*.
[One] should be careful and attentive, as this method is difficult to understand.

Commentary by Lín Lǐfēng 受業林禮豐按:

產後吸吸少氣，不能飲食者，病在太陽也。腹中刺痛不止，或苦少腹急摩痛引腰背者，病在厥陰也。病屬虛羸不足，故用桂枝湯倍芍，以助脾氣之輸；而刺痛牽引，乃血瘀滯著，故用當歸以通凝聚之瘀，使脾氣有權而得上輸下轉之力。故產後一月，日得服四五劑為善也。令人強壯宜者，得補益之功也。加飴糖者，以中土大虛，故用稼穡之味，以補中焦之氣血。若去血過多，崩傷內衄不止，則血海空虛，陰氣失守，故加地黃、阿膠之重濁味厚者以養陰。名之曰內補者，以產後虛羸，病偏於內也。古聖之方，無微不到，神乎！神乎！

Postpartum shortage of qì in spite of heavy inhalations with an inability to eat and drink, [means] that the disease is in tàiyīn.[111] Incessant stabbing pain in the abdomen or hypertonicity and pain in the lesser abdomen stretching to the lower back and back, [means] the disease is in juéyīn. [When] the disease belongs to vacuity emaciation and insufficiency, *Guì Zhī Tāng* with double *sháo yào* is used in order to assist the transportation [function] of spleen qì. Pulling and stabbing pain are due to blood stasis, therefore, *dāng guī* is used in order to free the congealing and gathering of stasis, giving spleen qì the power to transport upwards and move downwards. It is for this reason that it is very good to take four to five doses throughout the day over the first month after giving birth. This will provide women with strength as it has a supplementing and boosting effect. As for the addition of *yí táng*, [when] there is major vacuity of center earth, a sowing and reaping flavor is used in order to supplement the qì and blood of the center burner. If there is excessive blood loss, flooding, or incessant spontaneous internal bleeding, this means that the sea of blood is empty and vacuous, and yīn qì fails to keep to its abode; therefore, *dì huáng* and *ē jiāo's* heavy and thick flavors are added to nourish yīn. The name [of the formula] means to supplement the interior, for postpartum vacuity emaciation is primarily a disease of the interior. This formula of the ancient [medical] sage takes everything into account. Divine indeed! Divine indeed!

111. Although the original text says tàiyáng 太陽, I believe this is a typographical error, and should actually be tàiyīn 太陰.

婦人雜病方
Fù Nü Zá Bìng Fāng
Formulas for Miscellaneous Gynecological Diseases

小柴胡湯
Xiǎo Chái Hú Tāng
Minor Bupleurum Decoction

歌解見《傷寒》。

For the song with explanation, see the *Shāng Hán Lùn.*

治婦人中風，七八日續來寒熱，發作有時，經水適斷者，此為熱入血室，其血必結，故使如瘧狀，發作有時，此湯主之。

A treatment for women who have had wind strike for seven or eight days with alternating hot and cold at set times, and ceasing of menstruation. This indicates that heat has entered the blood chamber, and blood is bound, causing signs that resemble malaria, which occur at set times. This decoction rules it.

半夏厚朴湯
Bàn Xià Hòu Pò Tāng
Pinellia and Magnolia Bark Decoction

治婦人咽中如有炙臠者，此湯主之。

A treatment for women who feel as if there is a piece of fried meat in their throat. This decoction rules it.

半夏（ 一升 ）厚朴（ 三兩 ）茯苓（ 四兩 ）生薑（ 五兩 ）蘇葉（ 二兩 ）

bàn xià	半夏	200ml
hòu pò	厚朴	9g
fú líng	茯苓	12g
shēng jiāng	生薑	15g
sū yè	蘇葉	6g

上五味，以水一斗，煮取四升，分溫四服，日三夜一服。

Simmer the five ingredients above in 2,000ml of water until reduced to 800ml. Divide into four doses and take three throughout the day and one at night.

Song 歌曰:

狀如炙臠貼咽中，
卻是痰凝氣不通；
半夏一升茯四兩，
五兩生薑三兩厚朴二兩蘇葉攻。

The symptom of feeling as if a piece of fried meat were stuck in the throat
is due to congealed phlegm, and qì not moving freely;
200ml of *bàn xìa* and twelve grams of *fú líng*,
attacked with fifteen **grams** ***shēng*** *jiāng*, **nine grams** *hòu pò*, and six of *sū* ***yè***.

Commentary by [Chén] Yuánxī 男元犀按:

咽喉者，高之極；小腹者，下之極。炙臠貼於咽中者，病在上；奔豚起於小腹者，病在下；俱屬於氣，但其病有上下之分。蓋婦人氣鬱居多，或偶感客邪，依痰凝結，窒塞咽中，如有炙臠狀，即《千金》所謂咽中帖帖狀。吞之不下，吐之不出者，今人名曰梅核氣是也。主以半夏厚朴湯者，方中以半夏降逆氣，厚朴解結氣，茯苓消痰，尤妙以生薑通神明，助正祛邪，以紫蘇之辛香，散其鬱氣，鬱散氣調，而凝結焉有不化者哉？後人以此湯變其分兩，治胸腹滿悶嘔逆等證，名七氣湯，以治七情之病。

The throat is at the highest reaches [of the body], and the lower abdomen is at the lowest. [With] the feeling as if a piece of fried meat is stuck in the throat, the disease is in the upper body; with running piglet, which rises from the lower abdomen, the disease is in the lower body. Both diseases are related to qì; however the differentiation is based on whether the disease is in the upper or lower body. Women commonly suffer from qì depression. [With] contraction of visiting evil, [this evil] will combine with phlegm, which [then] congeals and obstructs the throat, resulting in the feeling as if a piece of fried meat were stuck [there]. This is described as stickiness in the throat in the *Qiān Jīn Fāng*. [This feeling of a piece of fried meat stuck in the throat] that can neither be vomited up nor swallowed down is what people nowadays refer to as plum pit qì. The ruling formula is *Bàn Xià Hòu Pò Tāng*, which contains *bàn xià* to downbear counterflow qì, *hòu pò* to resolve bound qì, *fú líng* to disperse phlegm, and the particularly ingenious *shēng jiāng*, which promotes the enlightenment of the spirit, and assists the right [qì] in expelling evil. The acrid and fragrant *sū yè* dissipates depressed qì, as once this depression is dissipated, qì will be regulated, and then how could the congealed and bound [phlegm] not be transformed? In later times, people have altered the dosages [and ingredients of the formula] in order to treat fullness and oppression in the chest and abdomen with retching counterflow, re-naming it *Qī Qì Tāng* [seven qì decoction] to treat diseases of the seven affects.

甘麥大棗湯

Gān Mài Dà Zǎo Tāng

Licorice, Wheat, and Jujube Decoction

治婦人臟燥，悲傷欲哭，象如神靈所作，數欠伸，此湯主之。

A treatment for visceral agitation in women, which manifests as frequent sorrow with a desire to cry, appearance as if possessed by spirits, and frequent yawning and stretching, this decoction rules it.

甘草（ 三兩 ）小麥（ 一升 ）大棗（ 十枚 ）

gān cǎo	甘草	9g
xiǎo mài	小麥	200ml
dà zǎo	大棗	10 pcs

上三味，以水六升，煮取三升，分溫三服。亦補脾氣。

Simmer the three ingredients above in 1,200ml of water until reduced to 600ml. Divide and take warm, three doses per day. It also supplements the spleen qì.

Song 歌曰:

婦人臟燥欲悲傷，
如有神靈太息長；
數欠伸。
小麥一升三兩草，
十枚大棗力相當。

Visceral agitation in women, with frequent sorrow and a desire to cry,
an appearance as if possessed by spirits, and long sighs.
Frequent yawning and stretching.
200ml of of *xiǎo mài* and nine grams of *gān cǎo*,
with twelve pieces of *dà zǎo*, is considerably strong.

Quotation by Wèi Niàntíng 魏念庭云:

世醫竟言滋陰養血，抑知陰盛而津愈枯，陽衰而陰愈燥。此方治臟燥大法也。

Common physicians all believe that [visceral agitation should be treated by] enriching yīn and nourishing the blood, yet are unaware that [with] yīn exuberance, fluids can be more desiccated, and [with] yáng debilitation, yīn can become more dry. The methods of this formula are a fundamental treatment for visceral agitation.

小青龍湯

Xiǎo Qīng Lóng Tāng

Minor Blue-Green Dragon Decoction

麻黃（三兩，去節）芍藥（三兩）五味子（半升）乾薑（三兩）甘草（三兩，炙）細辛（三兩）桂枝（三兩，去皮）半夏（半升，洗）

má huáng	麻黃	knots removed	9g
sháo yào	芍藥		9g
wǔ wèi zǐ	五味子		100ml
gān jiāng	乾薑		9g
gān cǎo	甘草	honey-fried	9g
xì xīn	細辛		9g
guì zhī	桂枝	bark removed	9g
bàn xià	半夏	washed	100ml

上八味，以水一斗，先煮麻黃，減二升，去上沫，內諸藥，煮取三升，去滓，溫服一升。

For the eight ingredients above use 2,000ml of water. First boil the *má huáng* and reduce the water by 400ml. Remove the foam collecting on the surface, and add the other ingredients. Boil until reduced to 600ml, remove the dregs, and take 200ml warm.

瀉心湯

Xiè Xīn Tāng

Heart Draining Decoction

治婦人吐涎沫，醫反下之，心下即痞。當先治其吐涎沫，小青龍湯主之；涎沫止，乃治痞，瀉心湯主之。

A treatment for women with ejection of foamy drool that was inappropriately precipitated, which immediately [manifests with] glomus below the heart. [One should] treat the ejection of foamy drool first, and *Xiǎo Qīng Lóng Tāng* rules it. Once the ejection of foamy drool has stopped, treat the glomus [for which] *Xiè Xīn Tāng* rules.

大黃（二兩）黃連黃芩（各一兩）

dà huáng	大黃	6g
huáng lián	黃連	3g
huáng qín	黃芩	3g

上三味，以水三升，煮取一升，頓服之。

Simmer the three ingredients above in 600ml of water until reduced to 200ml, and take by drinking in one gulp.

Commentary 按:

二方解見《傷寒論淺注》，不再釋。

The explanation for both formulas is seen in the *Shāng Hán Lùn Qiǎn Zhù*,[112] so there is no need for further explanation.

112. The *Shāng Hán Lùn Simply Annotated* by Chén Xiūyuán.

溫經湯

Wēn Jīng Tāng

Channel Warming Decoction

治婦人年五十所，病下利數十日不止，暮即發熱，少腹裏急，腹滿，手掌煩熱，唇口乾燥，此屬帶下。何以故？曾經半產，瘀血在少腹不去。何以知之？其證唇口乾燥，故知之，當以此湯主之。

A treatment for women in their fifties who suffer from incessant diarrhea more than ten times per day, with heat effusion in the evening, lesser abdominal urgency, abdominal fullness, vexing heat in the palms, and dry lips and mouth. This belongs to women's diseases. What is the reason? There was a history of late miscarriage and static blood now remains in the lesser abdomen. How can one know this? The pattern manifests with dry lips and mouth, and this is how one knows this, and this formula rules it.

吳茱萸（三兩）當歸芎藭芍藥人參桂枝阿膠丹皮甘草（各二兩）生薑（三兩。一本二兩）[113]半夏（半升。一本一升）[114]麥冬（一升）

wú zhū yú	吳茱萸	9g
dāng guī	當歸	6g
chuān xiōng	芎藭	6g
sháo yào	芍藥	6g
rén shēn	人參	6g
guì zhī	桂枝	6g
ē jiāo	阿膠	6g
dān pí	丹皮	6g
gān cǎo	甘草	6g
shēng jiāng	生薑	9g
bàn xià	半夏	100ml
mài dōng	麥冬	200ml

113. Another edition uses 6g.

114. Another edition uses 200ml.

上十二味，以水一斗，煮取三升，分溫三服 。亦主婦人少腹寒，久不受胎；兼治崩中去血，或月水來多，及至期不來 。

Simmer the eleven ingredients above in 2,000ml of water until reduced to 600ml. Divide and take warm in three doses. It also rules [the treatment] of lesser abdominal cold in women and infertility, and simultaneously treats flooding, copious menstruation, as well as delayed menstruation.

Song 歌曰:

溫經芎芍草歸人，
膠桂丹皮二兩均，八物各二兩。
半夏半升麥冬倍用，
生薑吳茱萸三兩對君陳 。

For *Wēn Jīng Tāng* [use] *chūan xiōng, sháo yào, gān cǎo, dāng guī, rén shēn, ē jiāo, guì zhī,* and *dān pí* at six grams each. **Six grams for each of the eight medicinals.**
Use 100ml of *bán xiá* and double of ***mài dōng,***
plus nine grams each of ***shēng*** *jiāng* and ***wú zhū*** *yú.*

Commentary by [Chén] Yuánxī 男元犀按:

方中當歸、芎藭、芍藥、阿膠，肝藥也；丹皮、桂枝，心藥也；吳茱萸，肝藥亦胃藥也；半夏，胃藥亦衝藥也；麥門冬、甘草，胃藥也；人參補五臟，生薑利諸氣也。病在經血，以血生於心，藏於肝也，衝為血海也。胃屬陽明，厥陰衝脈麗之也。然細繹方意：以陽明為主，用吳茱萸驅陽明中土之寒，即以麥門冬滋陽明中土之燥，一寒一熱，不使偶偏，所以謂之溫也；用半夏、生薑者，以薑能去穢而胃氣安，夏能降逆而胃氣順也；其餘皆相輔而成溫之之用，絕無逐瘀之品。故過期不來者能通之，月來過多者能止之，少腹寒而不受胎者並能治之，統治帶下三十六病，其神妙不可言矣。

Within the formula, *dāng guī, chūan xiōng, sháo yào,* and *ē jiāo* are all liver medicinals; *dān pí* and *guì zhī* are heart medicinals; *wú zhū yú* is both a liver and stomach medicinal; *bán xiá* is both a stomach and thoroughfare [vessel] medicinal; *mài dōng* and *gān cǎo* are stomach medicinals; *rén shēn* supplements the five viscera, and *shēng jiāng* disinhibits all qì. Disease is in the menstrual blood. Blood is engendered in the heart, stored in the liver, and the thoroughfare vessel is the sea of blood. The stomach belongs to yángmíng, and is linked[115] to both the juéyīn and the thoroughfare vessel. Now [we must] carefully examine the meaning of the formula. As [the condition] is ruled by yángmíng, *wú zhū yú* is used to expel cold from yángmíng center earth, while *mài dōng* enriches dryness within yángmíng center earth – one cold and one hot medicinal. [While being] neither too cold nor too warm, [the formula] is [still] referred to as warm. As for the usage of *bán xiá* and *shēng jiāng*: *shēng jiāng* eliminates foulness and calms stomach qì, while *bán xiá* is able to down-bear counterflow and smooth stomach qì. The remaining [medicinals] are used to assist in warming, and are by no means ingredients for expelling stasis. Therefore, with delayed menstruation [this formula] is able to free it, and with excessive menstruation it is able to stop it. It is [also] able to treat lower abdominal cold and infertility, and for the thirty-six women's diseases, its marvel is too wonderful for words!

115. Here the character *lí* 麗 implies connection, integration, or linkage.

土瓜根散

Tǔ Guā Gēn Sǎn

Thladiantha Powder

治帶下經水不利，少腹滿痛，經一月再見者，此散主之 。

A treatment for women's diseases with inhibited menstruation, fullness and pain in the lesser abdomen, and menses that appear twice a month. This powder rules it.

土瓜根芍藥桂枝蟅蟲（ 各三分 ）

tǔ guā gēn	土瓜根	3 parts
sháo yào	芍藥	3 parts
guì zhī	桂枝	3 parts
zhè chóng	蟅蟲	3 parts

上四味，杵為散，酒服方寸匕，日三服 。

Process the four ingredients above by pestling them into a powder. Take one gram with liquor, three doses per day.

Song 歌曰:

帶下端由瘀血停，
不能如期而至，
以致少腹滿痛。
月間再見既瘀而不行，
則前經未暢所行，
不及待後月正期而至，
故一見再見。
不循經；經， 常也。
言不循常期也。
蟅瓜桂芍均相等，
調協陰陽病自寧 。

Women's diseases are caused by stasis and stoppage.
[If the menses] is unable to arrive on schedule,
this results in lesser abdominal fullness and pain.
Menses appear twice a month. **Since there is stasis and lack of movement,**
[and] the previous menses could not move freely,
[the accumulated blood] does not wait [to come out] at the time of the normal cycle,
therefore, the menses appears twice in a month.
The menses [do not] follow the cycle, **the cycle [should be] regular.**
Therefore it means that [the menses] do not arrive on a regular basis.
Thus, equal parts of *zhè chóng, tǔ guā gēn, guì zhī,* and *sháo yào*
will harmonize yīn and yáng [and the] disease will quiet on its own.

Commentary by [Chén] Yuánxī 男元犀按:

此條單指經水不利之帶下病也。經者，常也。婦人行經，必有常期。尤云：血滿則行，血盡復生，如月之盈虧，海之潮汐，必定應期而至，謂之信。此云經水不利，一月再見者，乃蓄洩失常，則有停瘀之患也。然瘀既停，必著少腹之間作滿而痛也。立土瓜根散者，為調協陰陽，主驅熱通瘀之法。方中桂枝通陽，芍藥行陰，使陰陽和，則經之本正矣；土瓜根驅熱行瘀，蟅蟲蠕動逐血，去其舊而生新，使經脈流暢，常行不亂也。

This clause simply refers to inhibited menstruation in women's diseases. The character *jīng* [經] [also means] regular. [With] women, menstruation needs to occur in a regular cycle. Yóu Zàijīng said: when the blood is full, it moves, and when exhausted [it should] regenerate. [This is] similar to the waxing and waning of the moon, and the tides of the ocean, which are sure to arrive at their appointed time. This [line] says, 'inhibited menstruation, seen twice a month.' Only when storage and discharge are abnormal, then [one] suffers from stoppage and stasis. Stoppage and stasis will invariably result in fullness and pain in the lesser abdomen. *Tǔ Guā Gēn Sǎn* harmonizes yīn and yáng and rules the method of expelling heat and freeing stasis. Within the formula *guì zhī* frees yáng, and *sháo yào* moves yīn, bringing forth the harmony of yīn and yáng, which results in the regulation of the foundation of the menses. *Tǔ guā gēn* expels heat and moves stasis. *Zhè chóng* [causes] peristalsis in order to move the blood, expelling the old to engender the new, enabling the channel vessels to flow smooth and easy, moving regularly without disorder.

旋覆花湯

Xuán Fù Huā Tāng

Inula Decoction

歌見積聚。

For the formula, see [the section on] "Accumulations and Gatherings."

治婦人得革脈，則半產漏下 。

A treatment for women with scallion-stalk pulses, which indicates late miscarriages and spotting.

旋覆花（ 三兩 ）蔥（ 十四莖 ）新絳（ 少許 ）

xuán fù huā	旋覆花	9g
cōng	蔥	14 stems
xīn jiàng	新絳	a small amount

上三味，以水三升，煮取一升，頓服之 。

Simmer the three ingredients above in 600ml of water until reduced to 200ml, and take by drinking in one gulp.

Commentary by [Chén Yuán] Xī 犀按:

旋復花湯，《金匱》中兩見：一治積聚症，以通肝著之氣；一治婦人雜病症，以化弦芤為革之脈。若革脈不化，則必半產漏下，但此方非謂漏下時始用耳。

Xuán Fù Huā Tāng is seen twice in the *Jīn Guì Yào Lüè*; once to treat accumulations and gatherings by freeing the qì in liver stickiness, and again to treat miscellaneous women's diseases with pulses that have become wiry and scallion-stalk like. If the scallion-stalk pulses have not changed, then there will be late miscarriages and spotting. However, it is not suggested that [one] should only use this formula at the onset of spotting.

膠薑湯

Jiāo Jiāng Tāng

Ass Hide Glue and Ginger Decoction

方闕。或云：即是乾薑、阿膠二味煎服。林云：即是膠艾湯。千金膠艾湯亦可取用。

[This] formula is missing. Some have said that this is simply just *gān jiāng* and *ē jiāo* taken together as a decoction. Lín[116] says that this formula is *Jiāo Ài Tāng*. *Jiāo Ài Tāng* from the *Qiān Jīn Yì Fāng* can also be used.[117]

治婦人陷經、漏下黑不解者，主之。

A treatment for women with fallen menstruation and incessant spotting of dark blood, [this decoction] rules it.

Song 歌曰:

膠薑方闕症猶藏，
漏下陷經黑色詳；
薑性溫提膠養血，
剛柔運化配陰陽。

The formula *Jiāo Jiāng* [*Tāng*] is missing, but its related symptoms have been collected,
which are spotting and fallen menstruation of a black color;
the nature of *jiāng* is warm and lifting, while *ē jiāo* nourishes the blood.
Strong and supple to transport and transform both yīn and yáng.

116. Most likely referring to Lín Yì 林億 a *Sòng* Dynasty scholar-official who worked as a chief editor in the Bureau for Revising Medical Texts, editing most of the major classics prior to the *Táng* Dynasty.

117. The version of this formula in the *Qiān Jīn Yì Fāng* consists of *ē jiāo* 9g, *ài yè* 9g, *sháo yào* 9g, *gān dì huáng* 9g, *dāng guī* 9g, *gān jiāng* 6g, *chuān xiōng* 6g, and *zhì gān cǎo* 6g.

道光四年，閩都閫[118]府宋公，其三媳婦產後三月餘，夜半腹痛發熱，經血暴下鮮紅，次下黑塊，繼有血水，崩下不止，約有三四盆許，不省人事，牙關緊閉，挽余診之。時將五鼓矣。其脈似有似無，身冷面青，氣微肢厥。予曰：血脫當益陽氣。用四逆湯加赤石脂一兩，煎湯灌之，不差；又用阿膠、艾葉各四錢，乾薑、附子各三錢，亦不差。

In the fourth year of Dào Guāng[119] (1825), in the capital of Mǐn[120] at the official residence of a *Sòng* general, the third daughter-in-law who was in her third month following childbirth, had suffered from abdominal pain and heat effusion in the middle of the night. [In addition], she had sudden menstrual bleeding, which was fresh red, followed by black clots. She continued to have incessant flooding of watery-thin blood, and [lost] approximately three or four basins full. She had lost consciousness, [and had] a clenched jaw, at which point, I was called in for diagnosis. At that time it was already the fifth watch just before dawn. Her pulse would appear and disappear; she had a cold body with a greenish-blue complexion, faint breathing, and reversal cold. I said that with blood desertion, yáng qì needed to be boosted. I used *Sì Nì Tāng* with thirty grams of *chì shí zhī*, decocted and poured into her mouth. There was no response. I then used twelve grams each of *ē jiāo* and *ài yè*, with nine grams each of *gān jiāng* and *fù zǐ*, and she also failed to recover.

沉思良久，方悟前方用乾薑守而不走，不能導血歸經也，乃用生薑一兩，阿膠五錢，大棗四枚。服半時許，腹中微響，四肢頭面有微汗，身漸溫，須臾蘇醒，自道身中疼痛。余令先與米湯一杯，又進前方，血崩立止，脈復厥回。大約膠薑湯，即生薑、阿膠二味也。蓋阿膠養血平肝，去瘀生新，生薑散寒升氣，亦陷者舉之，鬱者散之，傷者補之，育之之義也。

I contemplated this for a while, and then realized that *gān jiāng* in the previous formula was more static than active, and would be unable to guide the blood back into the channels. Thereupon, I used thirty grams of *shēng jiāng*, fifteen grams of *ē jiāo*, and four pieces of *dà zǎo*. After taking about half of the decoction, her abdomen started making noises, and a slight sweat emanated from her limbs, head and face. Her body gradually started to get warm, and then she instantly regained consciousness. [Upon awakening] she said [she had] generalized body pain. I advised her to first take a cup of rice decoction, and [then] take the previous decoction [once again]. Afterwards her flooding immediately stopped, her pulse was restored, and the reversal was returned. [Therefore I believe] *Jiāo Jiāng Tāng* is probably only composed of two medicinals, *shēng jiāng* and *ē jiāo*. Now, *ē jiāo* nourishes the blood, calms the liver, eliminates stasis and engenders the new. *Shēng jiāng* dissipates cold, and ascends qì, so sinking can be lifted. [Therefore] the meaning [behind the formula] is to dissipate depression, supplement damage, and nourish.

118. The character *kǔn* 閫 here can be defined as city gate, but in addition, can also be translated as capital.

119. The reign name of the *Qīng* emperor (1821–1850).

120. An abbreviation for Fújiàn province.

大黃甘遂湯

Dà Huáng Gān Suì Tāng

Rhubard and Kansui Decoction

治婦人少腹滿如敦狀，小便微難而不渴，此為水與血俱結在血室也，此湯主之。

A treatment for women with lower abdominal fullness that resembles a *duì*,[121] with slight difficulty in urination and an absence of thirst. This is due to the binding of water and blood in the blood chamber, and this decoction rules it.

大黃（四兩）甘遂阿膠（各二兩）

dà huáng	大黃	12g
gān suì	甘遂	6g
ē jiāo	阿膠	6g

上三味，以水三升，煮取一升，頓服，其血當下。

Simmer the three ingredients above in 600ml of water until reduced to 200ml, and take by drinking in one gulp.

Song 歌曰:

小腹敦形
敦音對，古器也。
《周禮》槃以乘血，敦以乘食，
小腹高起之狀相似也。
小腹，胞之室也。
胞為血海，其滿大為蓄血也。
小水難，
小水難而不渴，亦蓄水也。
水同瘀血兩彌漫；結在血室。

121. A *duì* 敦 is an ancient vessel once used to hold millet, which was small on both ends and larger in the middle.

大黃四兩遂膠二，
頓服瘀行病自安。

The lower abdomen appears as if the shape of a *duì.*
***Duì* 敦 sounds the same as *duì* 對, and is an ancient receptacle.**
In the *Zhōulǐ*[122] a *pán*[123] was used to carry blood, while a *duì* was used to carry food.
The swelling of the abdomen here resembles a *duì*.
The lower abdomen is the chamber of the uterus.
The uterus is the sea of blood, and when full and large, this is blood amassment.
Difficult urination,
[when] urination is difficult with an absence of thirst, this is also water amassment;
[is a result of] the permeation of both water and static blood [which] **bind in the blood chamber.**
Twelve grams of *dà huáng* with six of *gān suì* and *ē jiāo,*
taken in one gulp [results in] the moving of stasis and the natural quieting of the disease.

Commentary by [Chén] Yuánxī 男元犀按:

方中大黃攻血蓄，甘遂攻水蓄，妙得阿膠本清濟之水，伏行地中，歷千裏而發於古東阿縣之井，此方取其以水行水之義也。《內經》謂：濟水內合於心。用黑驪皮煎造成膠，以黑屬於腎，水能濟火，火熄而血自生，此方取其以補為通之義也。然甘遂似當減半用之。

Within the formula, *dà huáng* attacks the blood amassment, *gān suì* attacks the water amassment, and the ingenuity lies in *ē jiāo,* which is [made] from the clear well water [of the] Jì [river], which moves deep within the earth. [The Jì river] passes a thousand miles [underground] and emerges in the ancient city of Dōng Ē. The idea behind this formula is to move water with water. The *Huáng Dì Nèi Jīng* says that the Jì river is interiorly related to the heart.[124] The skin of a black mule is decocted to create *ē jiāo,* and the color black is associated with the kidneys. Water is able to relieve fire, and when fire is extinguished, blood is engendered on its own. The intention of this formula is to use supplementation [in order to] free; therefore [one can] reduce the dosage of *gān suì* by half.

122. The *Zhōu Lǐ* 《周禮》(The Rites of Zhōu) is a seminal Confucian text dating back to the 2nd century BC.

123. An ancient washbasin.

124. The Jì River was used as a metaphor for the heart. It no longer exists, but was once part of the Yellow River (*huáng hé*), which originated in Jìyuán and Hénán and ran eastward to empty into the Bǒhǎi Bay. The lower portion of the river passed through Jǐnán city, which was so named for being south of the Jì River. This river dried up in the *Wèi-Jìn* period, sometime around 300 AD.

抵當湯
Dǐ Dàng Tāng
Resistance Decoction

歌解見《傷寒》。

For the song with explanation, see the *Shāng Hán Lùn.*

治婦人經水不利下者，主之。

A treatment for women with inhibited menstruation, [this decoction] rules it.

水蛭（ 二十個，熬 ）虻蟲（ 三十枚，熬 、去翅足 ）桃仁（ 二十個，去皮尖 ）大黃（ 三兩，酒浸 ）

shuǐ zhì	水蛭	boiled	20 pcs
méng chóng	虻蟲	boiled, wings and legs removed	30 pcs
táo rén	桃仁	remove the skin and tips	20 pcs
dà huáng	大黃	soaked in wine	9g

上四味，為末，以水五升，煮取三升，去滓，溫服一升 。

Process the four ingredients above into a powder, and simmer in 1,000ml of water until reduced to 600ml. Remove the dregs, and take 200ml warm.

Commentary by [Chén] Yuánxī 男元犀按:

婦人經水不利下，脈證俱實者，宜此方，否則當養其衝任之源。不可攻下。

This formula is suitable for women with inhibited menstruation whose pulse and pattern are both replete. Otherwise [in the absence of repletion] one should nourish the source of the thoroughfare and conception vessels, and not offensively precipitate.

礬石丸

Fán Shí Wán

Alum Pill

治婦人經水閉不利，臟堅癖不止，中有乾血，下白物者，主之。

A treatment for women with blocked or inhibited menstruation, incessant hard aggregation in the uterus with dry blood inside, and discharge of a white substance,[125] [this pill] rules it.

礬石（三分，燒）杏仁（一分）

fán shí	礬石	calcined	3 parts
xìng rén	杏仁		1 part

上二味末之，煉蜜為丸棗核大，內臟中，劇者再內之。

Process the two ingredients above into a powder and combine with refined honey, forming into pills the size of a jujube pit. Insert one pill into the vagina. In severe cases, insert another.

Song 歌曰:

經凝成癖閉而堅，
白物時流豈偶然？
蓄洩不時，胞宮生濕，
濕復生熱，所積之血，
轉為濕熱所腐，
而白物時時自下。
礬石用三分杏一分，
服時病去不遷延。

[When there is] congealing of the menses, which becomes blocked [with a] hard aggregation,
how can there be the occasional flowing of a white substance?
When the amassment periodically discharges, the uterus will generate dampness.

125. White vaginal discharge.

Dampness will in turn generate heat and the place in which it accumulates is the blood.
Dampness and heat then putrefy,
resulting in the frequent discharge of a white substance.
For when three parts *fán shí* and one of *xìng rén*
are taken the disease will be eliminated immediately without delay.

Quotation by Yóu Zàijīng 尤在涇云:

臟堅癖不止者，子臟乾血，堅凝成癖而不去也。乾血不去，則新血不榮，而經閉不利矣。由是蓄洩不時，胞宮生濕，濕復生熱；所積之血轉為濕熱所腐，而成白物，時時自下，是宜先去其臟之濕熱。礬石卻水除熱，合杏仁破結潤乾血也。

[When there is an] incessant hard aggregation with dry blood in the uterus, [this is due to] hardness that has accumulated and become an aggregation, which fails to leave. Dry blood is not eliminated, with the result that new blood is unable to flourish and [therefore] menstruation becomes blocked or inhibited. Due to the periodic discharging of the amassment, the uterus generates dampness, which in turn engenders heat. The place where the damp-heat accumulate is in the blood; the dry blood is corroded by the [dampness and heat], and becomes a white substance, which then frequently discharges. Here it is appropriate to first eliminate the visceral[126] dampness and heat. *Fán shí* eliminates both water and heat, and when combined with *xìng rén*, they are able to break bind and moisten dry blood.

126. Referring to the uterus.

紅藍花酒

Hóng Lán Huā Jiǔ

Carthamus Wine

治婦人六十二種風，腹中血氣刺痛者，主之。

A treatment for sixty-two kinds of wind in women with blood and qì stabbing pain in the abdomen, [this wine] rules it.

紅藍花（一兩）

hóng lán huā	紅藍花	3g

上一味，酒一大升，煎減半，頓服一半，未止，再服。

Simmer the ingredient above in 200ml of wine, until reduced by half. Take half in a single gulp; if there is no resolution, take again.

Song 歌曰:

六十二風義未詳，
腹中刺痛勢彷徨；
治風先要行其血，
一兩藍花酒煮嘗。

[The] meaning [behind] the sixty-two kinds of wind is unknown,
[but there is] abdominal stabbing pain, which has a tendency to linger.
[When] treating wind, [one must] first move the blood;
cook three grams *lán huā* in wine, and drink.

《淺注》引張隱庵《侶山堂類辨》甚妙，不再釋。

The *Jīn Guì Yào Lüè Qiăn Zhù* quotes Zhāng Yǐnān's discussion of the formula from his *Lú Shān Táng Lèi Biàn*,[127] which is excellent, so it is superfluous to explain it again.

127. *Distinguishing of Categories from the Lú Shān Táng* written by Zhāng Yǐn'ān (Zhāng Zhìcōng) in 1663.

當歸芍藥散

Dāng Guī Sháo Yào Sǎn

Chinese Angelica and Peony Powder

方歌見妊娠。

For the formula, see [the section on] "Pregnancy."

治婦人腹中諸疾痛者，此方主之。

A treatment for all types of abdominal pain in women, this formula rules it.

當歸（三兩）芍藥（一斤，一作六兩）[128]茯苓（四兩）白朮（四兩）澤瀉（半斤）芎藭（半斤，作三兩）[129]

dāng guī	當歸	9g
sháo yào	芍藥	48g
fú líng	茯苓	12g
bái zhú	白朮	12g
zé xiè	澤瀉	24g
chuān xiōng	川芎	24g

上六味，杵為散，取方寸匕，酒和，日三服。

Grind the six ingredients above into a fine powder, and take one gram with wine, three doses per day.

128. Another edition writes 18g.
129. Another edition writes 9g.

Commentary by [Chén Yuán] Xī 犀按:

婦人腹中諸疾痛者，不外氣鬱、血凝、帶下等症。用當歸芍藥散者，以肝為血海，遂其性而暢達之也。方中歸、藭入肝，解鬱以伸木；芍、澤散瘀而行水；白朮培土養木；妙在作散以散之，酒服以調之，協諸藥通氣血，調營衛，以順其曲直之性，使氣血和，鬱滯散，何患乎腹中諸疾痛不除？

Most types of abdominal pain in woman are [due to] nothing more than qì depression, congealed blood, and leukorrhea. *Dāng Guī Sháo Yào Sǎn* is used, as the liver is the sea of blood, and its nature is to smoothly outthrust. Within the formula, *dāng guī* and *chuān xiōng* enter the liver and resolve depression in order to stretch wood; *sháo yào* and *zé xiè* dissipate stasis and move water; *bái zhú* banks up earth to nourish wood; The ingenuity [of the formula] lies in the fact that a powder [散] is used to dissipate [散].[130] [The formula] is taken with wine in order to harmonize and assist all the medicinals in freeing the qì and blood, and regulating the nutritive and defense in order to normalize the nature of bending and straightening. [Once] qì and blood have been brought into harmony and depression and stagnation are dissipated, how can one not be relieved from the suffering of all types of abdominal pain?

130. This statement alludes to the fact that the character for both dissipate and powder is *sǎn* 散.

小建中湯

Xiǎo Jiàn Zhōng Tāng

Minor Center-Strengthening Decoction

歌解見《傷寒》。

For the song with explanation, see the *Shāng Hán Lùn*.

治婦人腹中痛，此主之。

A treatment for women with abdominal pain, this [formula] rules it.

桂枝（三兩，去皮）甘草（三兩，炙）大棗（十二枚）芍藥（六兩）生薑（三兩）膠飴（一升）

guì zhī	桂枝	bark removed	9g
gān cǎo	甘草	honey-fried	9g
dà zǎo	大棗		12 pcs
sháo yào	芍藥		18g
shēng jiāng	生薑		9g
jiāo yí	膠飴		200ml

上六味，以水七升，煮取三升，去滓，內膠飴，更上微火消解，溫服一升，日三服。

Simmer the six ingredients above in 1,400ml of water until reduced to 600ml. Remove the dregs, add the *jiāo yí*, and again place on low heat until [the *jiāo yí*] has melted. Take 200ml warm, three doses per day.

嘔家不可用建中湯，以甜故也。

[Patients] that frequently vomit cannot take *Jiàn Zhōng Tāng* as it is [too] sweet.

Commentary by [Chén] Yuánxī 元犀按：

婦人腹中痛主以建中湯者，其意在於補中生血，非養血定痛也。蓋血無氣不生，無氣不行，得建中之力，則中氣健運，為之生生不息，即有瘀痛者，亦可平之。

[The treatment of] women with abdominal pain is ruled by *Jiàn Zhōng Tāng*. The intention [behind this formula] is to supplement the center to engender blood, and not to nourish the blood to settle pain. Without qì, blood is unable to be engendered or move, and by forcefully strengthening the center, central qì will be able to fortify and transport with the ability of engendering life without end. Even if there is stasis pain, [this formula] can also calm it.

腎氣丸

Shèn Qì Wán

Kidney Qì Pill

治婦人病，飲食如故，煩熱不得臥，而反倚息，名曰轉胞，不得溺也。以胞系了戾。故致此病，此方主之。

A treatment for women's disease where eating and drinking is normal, [but there is] vexing heat with sleeplessness, and also propped breathing. This is called shifted bladder, [and manifests with] an inability to urinate. This disease is caused by twisted connections of the bladder, and this formula rules it.

乾地黃（八兩）山藥山茱萸（各四兩）茯苓丹皮澤瀉（各三兩）附子（一枚，炮）桂枝（一兩）

gān dì huáng	乾地黃		24g
shān yào	山藥		12g
shān zhū yú	山茱萸		12g
fú líng	茯苓		9g
dān pí	丹皮		9g
zé xiè	澤瀉		9g
fù zǐ	附子	blast-fried	1 pc
guì zhī	桂枝		3g

上八味末之，煉蜜和丸梧子大，酒下十五丸，加至二十丸，日再服。

Process the eight ingredients above into a powder and combine with refined honey to form pills the size of firmiana seeds. Swallow fifteen pills [per dose] with liquor, increasing the dosage to a maximum of twenty pills, two doses per day.

Song 歌曰:

溫經暖腎整胞宮，
丹澤苓三地八融，
四兩萸薯桂附一，
端教系正腎元充 。

Warm the channels, the kidneys, and the bladder.
Blend nine grams *dān pí*, *zé xiè*, and *fú líng* with twenty-four grams *dì huáng*.
[Plus] twelve grams of *shān zhū yú* and *shān yào* with three grams of *guì zhī* and one piece of *fù zǐ*
[for] the connections [will be] upright, and the origin of the kidneys full.

Commentary by [Chén] Yuánxī 男元犀按:

胞為血海，與膀胱並列於臍下，俱懸空之腑，其氣相通，全賴腎氣充溢於其間，其胞系乃正。若腎氣不充，則胞系了戾，胞系了戾，必不得溺矣。是病雖在胞，其權則專在腎也，故以腎氣丸主之。方中地黃、山藥固腎臟之陰，山茱萸、附子補腎臟之陽，桂枝化腑氣，茯苓行水道，妙在澤瀉形圓善轉，俾腎氣旺，則能充於胞而系自正，系正則小便不利者而可利矣。

The uterus is the sea of blood, and is located alongside the bladder below the umbilicus. They are both suspended bowels with their qì being interlinked. The bladder depends on overflow from kidney qì into this space in order to be regular. If kidney qì is not full, then this will cause twisted connections of the bladder system. With twisted connections of the bladder system, there is an inability to urinate. Although this disease is in the bladder, the power is specifically in the kidneys, and therefore *Shèn Qì Wán* rules it. Within the formula, *dì huáng* and *shān yào* secure the yīn of the kidney viscera; *shān zhū yú* and *fù zǐ* supplement the yáng of the kidney viscera; *guì zhī* transforms bowel qì; *fú líng* moves the waterways, and the ingenuity [of the formula] lies in *zé xiè* whose shape is round and is very good at conveying qì, so [when] the spleen and kidneys are effulgent, they are able to fill the bladder so the connections can be right on their own. When the connections are right, then urination will be uninhibited and able to be discharged.

又主虛勞腰痛、少腹拘急、小便不利者。以腰為腎之外腑，腎司開合，主骨髓，為作強之官，與膀胱相表裏。若少陰精氣虛，不能主骨，則腰痛；少陰陽氣虛，不能通腑，則少腹拘急，小便不利。本方補益真陰，蒸動水氣，使陰平陽秘，開合之樞自如，故能治虛勞之病，然小便自利者，不宜服之，以其滲洩而更劫陰也。

It also rules [the treatment of] vacuity taxation lumbar pain, hypertonicity in the lesser abdomen, and inhibited urination. The lower back is the external palace of the kidneys; the kidneys are the office in charge of opening and closing, and rule the bones and marrow. The kidneys stand in an exterior interior relationship with the bladder. If shàoyīn essential qì is vacuous, it is unable to rule the bones, resulting in lumbar pain; with shàoyīn yáng qì vacuity, there is an inability to free the bowels, resulting in hypertonicity of the lesser abdomen, and inhibited urination. This formula supplements and boosts true yīn, steams and moves water qì, allows for yīn to be calm and yáng to be sound and for the smooth opening and closing of the pivot. Therefore, [this formula] is able to treat vacuity taxation disease. Now with uninhibited urination, this formula is unsuitable, due to [its ability of] percolating and discharging, [which will] further plunder the yīn.

蛇床子散

Shé Chuáng Zǐ Sǎn

Cnidium Seed Powder

治婦人陰寒，溫陰中坐藥，此散主之。

[When] treating genital cold in females, use a suppository to warm the genitals, [and] this powder rules.

蛇床子

shé chuáng zǐ	蛇床子

上一味末之，以白粉少許和合，相得如棗大，綿裹內之，自然溫。

Process the ingredient above into a powder with a small amount of white powder,[131] forming into pills the size of a jujube. Wrap in gauze and insert; warmth will appear naturally.[132]

131. White powder here may be referring to either rice powder or lead powder.

132. This medicinal is used as a suppository, which is inserted into the vagina. Once it has been inserted, the vagina will spontaneously become warm.

狼牙湯
Láng Yá Tāng
Wolf's Bane Decoction

治少陰脈滑而數者，陰中即生瘡，陰中蝕瘡爛者，此湯洗之。

A treatment for slippery and rapid shàoyīn pulses, with sores in the vagina. For putrefying eroding sores in the vagina, wash with this decoction.

狼牙（三兩）

láng yá 狼牙 9g

上一味，以水四升，煮取半升，以綿纏箸如繭，浸湯瀝陰中，日四遍。

Simmer the ingredient above in 800ml of water until reduced to 100ml. Wrap silk fibers around a chopstick like a silkworm cocoon, soak in the decoction, and drip into the vagina, four times daily.

Song 歌曰:

胞寒外候見陰寒，
納入蛇床佐粉安，
此溫胞益陽外治之善法，
為腎氣丸之佐也。
更有陰中瘡蠹爛者，
乃濕熱不潔而生蠹也。
狼牙三兩洗何難？
除濕熱殺蟲，
如無狼牙草，
以狼毒代之。

Genital cold is the external symptom of uterine cold,
and powdered *shé chuáng zǐ* [mixed with white] powder should be inserted [into the vagina].
This is an excellent external treatment method for warming the uterus and boosting yáng,

which can be complemented by *Shèn Qì Wán*.
Furthermore, how can it be difficult [to treat] genital sores [hidden worms][133] and putrefecation,
generated by impure dampness and heat [hidden worms],
with a wash of nine grams *láng yá*?
[Use to] **eliminate damp-heat and kill worms,**
and if *láng yá cǎo* is unavailable,
substitute with *láng dú*.

133. The term hidden worms refers to illnesses related to parasites in food.

膏發煎
Gāo Fā Jiān
Lard and Human Hair Brew

歌見黄癉。

For the song, see [the section on] "Jaundice."

治胃氣下洩，陰吹而正喧，此谷氣之實也，此主之 。

A treatment for downward drainage of stomach qì, with vaginal flatulence characterized by an incessant loud sound; which is due to repletion of grain qì. This [formula] rules it.

陰吹，陰中出聲，如大便矢氣之狀。

Vaginal flatulence is a sound, that emanates from the vagina, similar to flatus associated with bowel movements.

小兒疳蟲蝕齒方

Xiǎo Ér Gān Chóng Shí Chǐ Fāng

Pediatric *Gǎn* Worm-Eaten Tooth Formula

雄黃葶藶

xióng huáng	雄黃
tíng lì	葶藶

上二味末之，取臘月豬脂，熔以槐枝，綿裹頭四五枝，點藥烙之 。

Process the two ingredients above into a powder, mixing with melted pork lard, [that has been] collected at the end of the lunar year. Dip four or five twigs of *huái zhī* wrapped in gauze in the medicine, light it and fumigate the affected tooth.

Song 歌曰:

忽然出此小兒方，
本治疳蟲蝕齒良；
葶藶雄黃豬脂點烙，
闕疑留與後推詳 。

Suddenly this formula for children appears.
This [formula] is excellent at treating *gǎn* worm-eaten teeth.
Cauterize with *tíng lì, xióng huáng,* and melted pork **lard**.
[Any] missing [information] and doubt is left for later [generations] to study and clarify.

Commentary by [Chén Yuán] Xī 犀按:

蟲有大小之別，隨生處而異其形，總不離於風火濕，挾厥陰之氣化所生也，小兒疳蟲病者，多由母氏乳少。

Worms are differentiated based on their sizes, and [their] shapes are differentiated according to the locations [in which] they are generated. In general, they are transformed from wind, fire, and dampness, which combine with the qì of juéyīn. *Gǎn* worm disease in children is mostly due to scant breast milk in the mother.

多飼以火燥乾糧助火之品，致小兒煩啼不已，動其心包之火，火動必熏灼於肝。蒸鬱從風木化而為蟲。夫蟲乃有情之物。食有情之血。亂有情之心臟，起伏無定，妖妄作祟。故其證煩熱多汗，面青腹脹，喜食辛燥之味。又有蝕蟲，其形不一，小者名寸白蟲，主風木之氣鬱於中土所生也；大者為蝕蟲，乃宿食所化也。

Copious feeding of hot and dry foods will reinforce fire, resulting in vexation and incessant crying in children. Stirring of the pericardium fire invariably fumes and scorches the liver. The steaming and depression of wind-wood is transformed [into] worms. The worms have an affinity for matter, [their] food interest is blood, and [they] disturb the heart. When the worms move up and down and are not calm, [they] exert a disturbing influence, and therefore, [we see] signs of vexation heat, copious sweating, green-blue complexion, abdominal distention, and a craving for acrid and drying foods. Also, with erosion worms,[134] their appearances can vary; small ones are called inch white worms, which are mainly caused by wind and wood qì depression in center earth, and large ones are called food worms, which are the result of the transformation of abiding food.

有下蝕者，本心包之火協三焦蘊熱而成，著於前後二陰，名曰陰蝕，小如線，色白，抑或濕熱下注，兼以房事相侵，致陰中蝕爛，名曰蝕瘡。三者皆能使人咽乾而陰中痛痒。

Food worms in the lower body are caused by original pericardium fire assisting the triple burner in brewing heat, which becomes fixed in the anterior and posterior yīn and is referred to as yīn [genital] erosion. The smaller ones are like a thread and white in color, and may combine with downpouring damp-heat, and invade during sexual intercourse, causing erosion of the genitals, which are referred to as erosion sores. All three are capable of causing dryness of the throat and genital pain and itching.

有蝕齒者，生於齒縫齒齦，小如絲發，疼痛難忍，或名齒蛇，或名牙疳，能穿肉入骨。此症本於外感未解，邪火協心火薰灼而成。有小魚蟲者，如盆魚子初生之小，有兩目，有生足者，有無足者，吐出時如魚子動游狀，此乃胸氣不布，痰飲協木氣所生，故肝著症久而不愈，多生紅蝕。

134. Chén makes a note in this passage which says erosion [worms] are food worms.

Tooth erosion is engendered in the crack of the tooth and in the gums. It is small, resembling a silk thread, with pain that is difficult to endure. This is referred to as tooth snake or tooth *gǎn*, which can pass through the flesh and enter the bone. The root of this pattern is an unresolved exterior contraction, with fire evil assisting heart fire in fumigating and scorching. When there are small fish worms as small as basin fish eggs – where some have two eyes, some have feet and others do not – on vomiting there will be the appearance of small fish stirring and swimming. This is due to chest qì not spreading and phlegm-rheum assisting wood qì, resulting in a pattern of liver stickiness [which] is unresolved for an extended period of time, and engenders red erosion.

亦有眼目多壞，有鼠婦蟲者，形如小鼠婦，背有鱗甲，色微赤，有頭足眼目，吐出能跳躍，此受惡濁異氣、酒性鬱怒合化而生。然蟲症雖多，而仲師之方未有不備也。

Wood louse-like worms can ruin the eyes. [These] look like small wood louse, with scaly backs, which are slightly red in color and have heads, legs, and eyes. When vomited, they jump around. They are [due to] the contraction of foul pestilent qì, [which has] transformed from the combination of liquor, depression and anger. Nevertheless, even though worm patterns are numerous, the formulas of Master Zhàng are prepared [to deal with them].

今舉小兒疳病治法，意以補土清金，使天氣降而熱氣消，則土潤葉茂矣。

Now, using the treatment method for *gǎn* disease in children as an example, the idea is to supplement earth and clear metal, enabling heavenly qì to descend and hot qì to disperse so the earth can be moistened and the leaf[135] luxuriant.

近醫知為疳病，不辨寒熱實虛，多用毒藥殺蟲，而不知其愈殺愈生也，本方用雄黃、葶藶、豬脂、槐枝，主通氣行血之品，點藥烙之，如打摩之法，去積聚，調氣血，點之亦即熏之之法也。後人有神照法，從內經馬膏桑鉤方及此方套出。

Physicians nowadays are aware of *gǎn* disease, [yet] do not identify [between] cold and heat, or repletion and vacuity, and commonly use toxic medicinals to kill worms. [These physicians] are unaware that with more killing, there will be more generation. This formula uses *xióng huáng, tíng lì, zhū zhī,* and *huái zhī,* which are qì freeing, blood moving medicinals. The medicinals are applied through cauterization, similar to a method of a striking massage, in order to eliminate ac-

135. 'Leaf' here is used as a methaphorical reference to the lungs.

cumulations and gatherings, and regulate qì and blood. [Here] cauterization is used as a fumigation method. Later generations [derived] the *Shén Zhào* method[136] from the *Nèi Jīng's Mǎ Gāo Sāng Goū Fāng*[137] and this formula.

136. This *Shén Zhào* method, may be referring to the *shén dēng zhào fǎ* 神燈照法, a form of fumigation used to treat swelling and ulceration on the skin. The *Qīng* Dynasty physician Chéng Shānlíng 程山齡 said that with all swelling in the head it is inappropriate to use moxibustion out of fear of drawing fire qì upwards, and thus this form of fumigation is used instead.

137. This is referring to the formula *Mǎ Gāo Shēng Sāng Guì Jiǔ Fāng* 馬膏生桑桂酒方 mentioned in the *Huáng Dì Nèi Jīng*, which consists of *mǎ gāo*, *shēng sāng huī*, *guì zhī*, and *bái jiǔ*.

Appendix

Formulas, Indications, and Actions

Excerpted from the 1921 edition of the *Zhōng guó yī xué dà cí diǎn* 中國醫學大辭典 (Great Dictionary of Medicine in China) and arranged in the order in which the formulas occur in the source text.

旋覆花湯
Xuán Fù Huā Tāng

xuán fù huā	旋覆花	9g
cōng	蔥	14 stems
xīn jiàng	新絳	small amount

Indications: Treats liver stickiness where the patient frequently desires to pound on their chest. Before the acute stage only hot drinks are desired. In addition, it treats vacuity wind attacking the bladder in pregnant women, late miscarriages and spotting, with wiry, large, and scallion-stalk pulses.

Analysis:
- The nature of *xuán fù huā* is to convey qì downwards.
- *Cōng bái* is able to dissipate binds and dispel wind.
- The assistant *jiǎn sī* (natural silk) specifically supplements the bladder, and when dyed indigo-red is excellent for reaching the deep channels in order to dissipate bound qì.

麻仁丸
Má Rén Wán

má zǐ rén	麻子仁	400ml
sháo yào	芍藥	24g
zhǐ shí	枳實	24g
dà huáng	大黃	48g
hòu pò	厚朴	1 foot
xìng rén	杏仁	200ml

Indications: Treats a straitened spleen.

Analysis:
- A floating pulse indicates yáng exuberance, while a rough pulse indicates damage to yīn.
- If there is yáng exuberance and yīn damage, then there is desiccation of intestinal fluids, which are difficult to transport. This causes copious, frequent urination and constipation, and is referred to as a straitened spleen.
- Within the formula *má zǐ rén* is the sovereign with its copious fat content.
- *Xìng rén's* sweetness emolliates and serves as the minister.
- *Zhǐ shí* and *hòu pò* serve as the assistants and are able to normalize the qì and move stagnation.
- *Dà huáng's* role as the courier is to drain heat and precipitate.
- In addition, preparing this formula in pill form with refined honey moderates and moves, therefore causing the strength of the medicinals to remain within the intestines, as well as removing the heat and returning the fluids. From this the stools can be unobstructed.
- However, this formula is more appropriate in repletion patterns. In cases of constitutional vacuity, old age, or desiccated, and scanty blood, this formula cannot be given for it still may be too harsh and drying.

甘薑苓白朮湯
Gān Jiāng Líng Bái Zhú Tāng

gān cǎo	甘草	6g
bái zhú	白朮	6g
gān jiāng	乾薑	12g
fú líng	茯苓	12g

This formula is referred to as *Gān Cǎo Gān Jiāng Líng Zhú Tāng* in the *Jīn Guì Yào Lüè* and is also known as *Shèn Zhuó Tāng.*

Indications: Treats kidney stickiness disease.

Analysis:

- Here cold and damp are not located in the kidney viscera, but in the external dwelling of the kidneys.
- Therefore, treatment need not involve warming the kidneys in order to dissipate cold, but warming the earth in order to prevail over water.
- If *guì zhī* or *fù zǐ* were used, then kidney yīn would be damaged.

苓桂朮甘湯
Líng Guì Zhú Gān Tāng

fú líng	茯苓	12g
guì zhī	桂枝	9g
bái zhú	白朮	9g
gān cǎo	甘草	6g

Indications: Treats cold damage following ejection or precipitation with counterflow fullness below the heart, qì surging upwards into the chest, dizziness upon rising, a deep and tight pulse, and if sweating is promoted, there will be stirring of the channels, as well as quivering and trembling. It also treats phlegm-rheum below the heart with propping fullness in the chest and rib-sides and dizzy vision.

Analysis:

- This formula treats a pattern of upward surging of liver qì following ejection or precipitation. Ejection and precipitation have damaged the fluids of the spleen and stomach allowing for the exploitation of liver qì.
- It is known that in diseases of the liver, the spleen must first be replenished. This is the reason *guì zhī* is used in the formula, so as to treat the liver.
- The three medicinals *bái zhú, fú líng*, and *gān cǎo* supplement the spleen. When the spleen is weak it is unable to transport and fails to dam water. The result is the pervading of phlegm-rheum in the chest and rib-sides. Sovereign yáng becomes concealed, and rheum steeps into the branch collaterals resulting in propping fullness of the chest and rib-sides. This manifests with symptoms of vertigo, visual veiling dizziness, and palpitations.
- The formula uses *fú líng* to move the water of the spleen and lungs, *guì zhī* to vitalize heart yáng, *bái zhú* to supplement center earth, and *gān cǎo* to assist the spleen qì in its movement, as well as to promote interaction between the upper and lower body. Water will then have the power to descend downwards and not ascend and encroach the upper body.

腎氣丸
Shèn Qì Wán

gān dì huáng	乾地黃	24g
shān yào	山藥	12g
shān zhū yú	山茱萸	12g
zé xiè	澤瀉	9g
mǔ dān pí	牡丹皮	9g
fú líng	茯苓	9g
guì zhī	桂枝	3g
fù zǐ	附子	3g

Indications: Treats vacuity taxation with lumbar pain. Also treats dispersion-thirst with increased urination in men and shifted bladder with inability to urinate in women.

Analysis:
- *Shú dì* and *shān yào* enrich kidney yīn.
- *Shān zhū yú* and *fù zǐ* strengthen kidney yáng.
- *Guì zhī* transforms visceral qì.
- *Fú líng* promotes movement in the waterways.
- *Dān pí* and *zé xiè* eliminate toxic matter from within the blood and support the kidney in its task of qì transformation. Hence reducing the increased urination and freeing blockage.
- When the essence blood of the kidney viscera is full, then vacuity detriment is eliminated and lumbar pain will cease.

甘遂半夏湯
Gān Suì Bàn Xià Tāng

gān suì	甘遂	3 pcs
bàn xià	半夏	12 pcs
sháo yào	芍藥	5 pcs
gān cǎo	甘草	1 pc

Indications: Treats a hidden pulse, spontaneous diarrhea with gratification following the diarrhea, thirst, and continuous hardness, and fullness below the heart.

Analysis:
- Although there is diarrhea, there continues to be hardness and fullness below the heart.
- Rheum, which has not yet been terminated, pours below the heart.
- However, although the rheum has not yet been completely expelled, *gān suì's* offensive flushing and *bàn xià's* acrid dissipating functions are used to provide the momentum to guide it out.
- *Gān suì* and *gān cǎo* when used together are traditionally known to clash with one another. Therefore, in order to successfully dredge rheum one must drink a harsh formula.
- *Gān cǎo, sháo yào,* and honey are an ingenious combination used together to engender fluids, harmonize the center, and moderate the toxic medicinals.

十棗湯
Shí Zǎo Tāng

yuán huā	芫花	equal amounts
gān suì	甘遂	
dà jǐ	大戟	

Indications: Treats tàiyáng wind strike where the exterior has resolved and the interior is not yet harmonized. It also treats suspended and propping-rheum or cough due to water.

Analysis:
- *Yuán huā, gān suì,* and *dà jǐ* are all acrid-cold and toxic. They are powerful medicinals that flush and disinhibit.
- There is stoppage of water-rheum, which accumulates in the space between the channels and collaterals of the chest and diaphragm. Without *Shí Zǎo Tāng,* this cannot be eliminated.
- One must consider that this fierce and harsh method of treatment may damage the stomach, therefore *dà zǎo* is the sovereign.

- However, if original qì is not substantial, this formula must not be frivolously used.

大青龍湯
Dà Qīng Lóng Tāng

má huáng	麻黃	18g
guì zhī	桂枝	6g
gān cǎo	甘草	6g
xìng rén	杏仁	14 pits
shēng jiāng	生薑	9g
dà zǎo	大棗	10 pcs
shí gāo	石膏	1 pc the size of a chicken egg

Indications: Treats both tàiyáng wind and cold damage, and diseases of construction and defense manifesting with an absence of sweat, vexation, and agitation.

Analysis:

- Wind is treated with only *guì zhī*.
- Cold is treated with only *má huáng*.
- This formula is created by combining both *Guì Zhī Tāng* and *Má Huáng Tāng*, and thus simultaneously treats wind-cold and cold damage.
- As there is an absence of sweating in both patterns, there is no need for bitter, downbearing, and astringing *sháo yào*.
- As both patterns manifest with vexation and agitation, acrid cold *shí gāo* is used to resolve heat.
- In the event that there is an absence of vexation and agitation, one can still deal with this pattern by administering *Má Huáng Guì Zhī Gè Bàn Tāng*.
- When there is vexation and agitation in a *Dà Qīng Lóng Tāng* pattern, the heat is in both the flesh and the interior.
- At the initial stages of this tàiyáng pattern *shí gāo* is used as its acridity is able to resolve heat in the flesh, and its coldness can clear stomach fire. Its sweet flavor is able to generate liquids and humors, and is the first thing given to protect the fluids in yángmíng.
- If one is doubtful and fears using *shí gāo*, this will invariably result in the binding of heat in yángmíng, and can manifest with various signs such as macules, yellowing, mania, and muddledness.
- By observing all these facts, one can clearly understand that *shí gāo* is a very important medicinal for the treatment of cold damage and wind strike.

小青龍湯
Xiǎo Qīng Lóng Tāng

má huáng	麻黃	9g
sháo yào	芍藥	9g
wǔ wèi zǐ	五味子	100ml
gān jiāng	乾薑	9g
gān cǎo	甘草	9g
xì xīn	細辛	9g
guì zhī	桂枝	9g
bàn xià	半夏	100ml

Indications: Treats cold damage with an unresolved exterior, water qì below the heart, coughing, rapid panting, distention of the lung, chest fullness, nasal congestion and runny nose. In addition, there may also be coughing counterflow, propped breathing, and an inability to lie down.

Analysis:

- This formula treats cold damage tàiyáng disease with an unresolved exterior and moves interior water.
- In tàiyáng disease with stoppage of rheum, there are two kinds: the first is a wind strike exterior vacuity pattern with sweating, and is a *Wǔ Líng Sǎn* pattern; the second is cold damage exterior repletion with an absence of sweating, and this is a *Xiǎo Qīng Lóng Tāng* pattern.
- In an exterior repletion pattern with an absence of sweating, a dual *má huáng* and *guì zhī* formula can be given to resolve the exterior.
- *Dà zǎo* is removed, as its nature is cloying.
- *Xìng rén* is removed, as there is no panting. In the presence of panting, one can add it and would remove *shēng jiāng*, replacing it with *gān jiāng*.
- In the presence of retchingm *gān jiāng* and *xì xīn* are used to warmly dissipate. This causes the expulsion of cold and water out through the sweat.
- The assistant *bàn xià* expels phlegm in order to clear incessant fluids.
- *Wǔ wèi zǐ* assists by astringing the lung in order to restrain the consumption of damaged qì.
- The formula removes *bàn xià* and adds *huā fěn* to avoid dryness and generate fluids.
- *Má huáng* and *guì zhī* expel exterior evil out through tàiyáng.
- *Xì xīn* enters shàoyīn and moves interior water.
- *Gān jiāng* dissipates fullness in the front of the chest.
- *Bàn xià* downbears counterflow ascent of qì.
- In addition, when combining sour *wǔ wèi zǐ* with bitter *sháo yào*, the objective of using sour and bitter to eject and discharge is met. This results in downward movement, and *gān cǎo* is added to moderate it.
- Thoughtful consideration is given to these medicinals, and thus the location of evil qì and water-rheum is penetrated and attacked.
- All formless evil qì is expelled out through the fleshy exterior, while formed water-rheum is expelled out through the waterways. As a result both evil qì and water-rheum are cleared.
- Yù Jiāyán said: The significance behind the name *Xiǎo Qīng Lóng Tāng* is that the dragon is able to reach the storm, calming the waves and returning the rivers and sea. One does not want the water [of the earth] to ascend to the heavens, to generate clouds and produce excessive rain.
- If there is mild diarrhea, dysphagia, inhibited urination, and fullness in the lower abdomen, *má huáng* is removed, as this medicinal rules effusion and dissipation.
- Therefore, there is more emphasis on the interior and less so in the exterior.
- *Ráo huā*[1] is added to disinhinbit water, as once water is removed the diarrhea will stop on its own.

1. The flower of Wikstroemia canescens. In the *Shén Nóng Běn Cǎo Jīng* 《神農本草經》, this medicinal is said to be bitter and cold, and rules the treatment of cold damage, warm malaria evils, precipitates the twelve kinds of water, breaks accumulations, gatherings, large concretions and conglomerations, sweeps intestinal aggregations, food and drink accumulations, hot and cold evil qì, and disinhibits the water ways.

- Dysphagia is the result of the contention of water and cold qì in the exterior, and therefore *fù zǐ* is added in order to warm the center and as such the dysphagia will cease.
- Inhibited urination and fullness in the lower abdomen are due to the presence of water in the lower and not the upper, and so *fú líng* is used to disinhibit water. Once the urination is free the fullness will be gone.
- This formula and *Yuè Bì Tāng* both treat water-rheum spilling into the exterior. This manifests with distention in the skin and water swelling; it is appropriate here to effuse sweat in order to resolve the exterior. The only difference being that *Yuè Bì Tāng* treats heat and uses *shí gāo* as the sovereign in order to dissipate yáng water, while this formula treats cold by using *gān jiāng* and *guì zhī* in order to disperse yīn water.

木防己湯
Mù Fáng Jǐ Tāng

mù fáng jǐ	木防己	9g
shí gāo	石膏	2 pcs (the size of a large chicken egg)
guì zhī	桂枝	6g
rén shēn	人參	12g

Indications: Treats propping-rheum, manifesting with panting, fullness, glomus and hardness below the heart, a soot-black facial complexion, and a deep-tight pulse. This can last for several days and does not resolve following ejection or purgation.

Analysis:

- Within the formula *fáng jǐ* enters the hand tàiyīn lung channel. The lungs rule qì, and when qì transforms water moves on its own.
- *Guì zhī* enters the foot tàiyáng bladder channel. The bladder rules water, and when water moves qì spontaneously transforms.
- The combination of these two medicinals, one acrid and one bitter inevitably moves water qì dissipating the bind. Once water moves, the bind dissipates and the hard glomus below the heart is eliminated.
- Since the disease has lasted for more than several tens of days and ejection and purgation have been used, it is known that stomach yīn is damaged, and vacuous qì is running counterflow.
- Therefore, *rén shēn* is used in order to generate the already damaged yīn.
- *Shí gāo* is used to suppress the vacuous counterflow of qì.
- Once yīn is returned to a balanced state, the panting, fullness, and soot-black facial complexion will spontaneously resolve.

木防己去石膏加茯苓芒硝湯
Mù Fáng Jǐ Qù Shí Gāo Jiā Fú Líng Máng Xiāo Tāng

mù fáng jǐ	木防己	9g
guì zhī	桂枝	6g
fú líng	茯苓	12g
rén shēn	人參	12g
máng xiāo	芒硝	60ml

Indications: Treats propping-rheum in the diaphragm. Taken if *Mù Fáng Jǐ Tāng* offered no relief.

Analysis:

- *Mù Fáng Jǐ Tāng* utilizes *guì zhī* and *shí gāo*, one acrid-warm and one acrid-cool medicinal in order to course the lung. However they are not able to break hardness, so are therefore used to treat at the onset of the formation of propping-rheum.

- Once rheum evil has endured for an extended period of time, qì and blood will intertwine and form hard binds.
- Without adding *fú líng* with its bland percolation function, or *máng xiāo* with its ability to break and disinhibit, one would be unable to eliminate the bind.
- Therefore, it is said that in this case, using hardness to cast away hardness would not break it, but instead one should use softness to dispose of hardness.

澤瀉湯
Zé Xiè Tāng

zé xiè	澤瀉	15g
bái zhú	白朮	6g

Indications: Treats propping-rheum below the heart, where the person suffers from veiling dizziness.

Analysis:

- The heart is yáng within yáng.
- The head is the gathering place of all yáng.
- When there is propping-rheum below the heart, water-rheum will ascend and cloud the heart obstructing heart yáng. The yáng is then unable to gather at the top of the head, and therefore, one suffers from dizziness and dizzy vision.
- Within the formula, *zé xiè* is the sovereign. This guides the qì of water yīn in its downward movement, and discharges propping-rheum evil.
- However, with fear of water rising again after it has descended, the sweet and warm assistant *bái zhú* is used. Earth can restrain the various forms of water, so while still treating water, an embankment is built.

厚朴大黃湯
Hòu Pò Dà Huáng Tāng

hòu pò	厚朴	1 foot
dà huáng	大黃	18g
zhǐ shí	枳實	4 pcs

Indications: Treats propping-rheum with chest fullness.

Analysis:

- There are various types of propping-rheum.
- The chest is the pathway of yáng qì.
- Rheum is a yīn evil.
- When we say "chest fullness" this is due to yīn occupying the position of yáng, and filling the chest with cold causing fullness.
- The sovereign is *hòu pò*, which is bitter in flavor, warm in nature, and works on the qì level. *Hòu pò's* bitter flavor descends, while it's warmth opens, thus freeing the yáng qì, and transforming rheum in the chest.
- *Zhǐ shí* is round in shape, and aromatic in fragrance. The fragrance awakens the spleen, and its roundness rules rotation; therefore it is used as the assistant.
- *Dà huáng* is used to directly clear the pathway.
- Once this path is free, how can rheum evil not have a favorable flow in order to be eliminated downwards?

葶藶大棗瀉肺湯
Tíng Lì Dà Zǎo Xiè Fèi Tāng[2]

小半夏湯
Xiǎo Bàn Xià Tāng

bàn xià	半夏	200ml
shēng jiāng	生薑	24g

Indications:
1) Treats propping-rheum and phlegm accumulation above the diaphragm with panting, coughing, vomiting, and hiccup.
2) Treats jaundice, where the color of the urine is unchanged, with a desire to spontaneously discharge, abdominal fullness, and panting.

Analysis:
- In the formula, the key point is the use of acrid *shēng jiāng* to dissipate propping-rheum.
- *Bàn xià* is warm, downbears counterflow, and calms the stomach.
- Together these two medicinals serve to flush away rheum and cause downward movement.
- In jaundice where the color of the urine is unchanged with desire to naturally disinhibit, it is known that there is no static heat in the interior.
- Therefore, *bàn xià* is used to harmonize the stomach in order to settle counterflow.
- *Shēng jiāng* warms the interior central viscera.
- Once the center is warm, the functions of upbearing and downbearing are unobstructed. Thus, panting, fullness, retching, and counterflow will resolve on their own.

2. Refer to page 169 of volume 1.

己椒藶黄丸
Jǐ Jiāo Lì Huáng Wán

fáng jǐ	防己	3g
jiāo mù	椒目	3g
tíng lì	葶藶	3g
dà huáng	大黄	3g

Indications: Treats abdominal fullness with thirst, and a dry mouth and tongue, indicating water qì in the intestines.

Analysis:
- In this formula *fáng jǐ* and *jiāo mù* both guide rheum out through the front by the way of the urine.
- *Dà huáng* and *tíng lì* push rheum out through the back by the way of the bowels.
- Once separately eliminated through both ends, abdominal fullness is reduced and water-rheum moves.
- Subsequently, spleen qì is able to move and generate liquids and humors.

小半夏加茯苓湯
Xiǎo Bàn Xià Jiā Fú Líng Tāng

bàn xià	半夏	200ml
shēng jiāng	生薑	24g
fú líng	茯苓	12g

Indications: Treats phlegm-rheum with copious sweating, inhibited urination, sudden vomiting and retching, and glomus below the heart. These symptoms indicate stoppage of water in the chest and diaphragm, along with dizziness.

Analysis:

- Stagnant water below the heart causes glomus.
- Water intimidating the heart causes dizziness and palpitations.
- Water obstructing the chest and diaphragm inhibits the upbearing and downbearing mechanism of yīn and yáng and causes vomiting.
- This formula uses *bàn xià* to downbear counterflow, *shēng jiāng* to disinhibit qì, and *fú líng* to abduct water.
- This combination is an effective prescription to flush out phlegm, and stabilize vomiting.

五苓散
Wǔ Líng Sǎn

zé xiè	澤瀉	3.75g
zhū líng	豬苓	2.25g
fú líng	茯苓	2.25g
bái zhú	白朮	2.25g
guì zhī	桂枝	1.5g

Indications: Treats heat in the water aspect with inhibited urination and vexing thirst. Also treats the internal stoppage of water-rheum with palpitations below the umbilicus.

Analysis:

- This is a major formula that treats inhibited urination due to water and heat.
- The sovereign *zé xiè* is salty and cold and can penetrate the storehouse of water and discharge evil heat.
- The ministers *fú líng* and *zhū líng* are bland percolators, which free the waterways, and discharge water and heat.
- The assistant *bái zhú* is bitter, drying and can fortify and strengthen spleen earth in order to transport water.
- The courier *guì zhī* is acrid, warm and is able to steam and transform the triple burner in order to move water.
- When *zé xiè* is used with *fú líng* and *zhū líng*, then the downbearing and water disinhibiting strength is increased.
- When *bái zhú* is combined with *guì zhī*, then the upbearing and freeing of yáng effect is achieved swiftly.
- If one desires to effuse and dissipate exterior evil, then use *guì zhī* with hot drinks.
- If one desires to resolve vacuity cold in the bladder, then use *roù guī* with hot drinks.
- If one desires to disinhibit urination, use cold drinks, and this increases the strength of *zé xiè*. However, if there is a desire to vomit, use warm drinks.
- Do not erroneously administer hot drinks in patterns of yīn vacuity where the springs have dried out.

《外臺》茯苓飲
Wài Tái Fú Líng Yǐn

fú líng	茯苓	9g
rén shēn	人參	9g
bái zhú	白朮	9g
zhǐ shí	枳實	6g
jú pí	橘皮	7.5g
shēng jiāng	生薑	12g

The formula is originally from the *Wài Tái Mì Yào Fāng*.

Indications: Treats collected phlegm and abiding water in the heart and chest with vacuity of the heart, fullness of qì, and an inability to eat following the spontaneous vomiting of water.

Analysis:

- When the spleen and stomach are vacuous, they are unable to transport and transform, therefore this formula uses medicinals to strengthen and supplement the stomach.
- *Bái zhú* fortifies the spleen.
- *Fú líng* disinhibits dampness.
- *Chén pí* moves water.
- *Zhǐ shí* dissipates fullness.
- *Shēng jiāng* frees yáng.
- As a result the spleen and stomach are moved and fortified and vacuity fullness is dissipated.
- When there is still stoppage of rheum, even though *zhǐ shí* and *jú pí* are able to move this, *rén shēn* and *bái zhú* can complicate the stagnation of the phlegm-rheum, therefore, the formula cannot be used.

十棗湯
Shí Zǎo Tāng

See above.

小青龍湯
Xiǎo Qīng Lóng Tāng

See above.

桂苓五味甘草湯
Guì Líng Wǔ Wèi Gān Cǎo Tāng

guì zhī	桂枝	12g
fú líng	茯苓	12g
wǔ wèi zǐ	五味子	100ml
gān cǎo	甘草	9g

Indications: A treatment for when after taking *Xiǎo Qīng Lóng Tāng* there is copious spittle, a dry mouth, a deep pulse at the inch opening and a faint pulse at the cubit position. The patient has reverse counterflow in the hands and feet, qì surging up from the lower abdomen to the chest and throat, impediment in the extremities, a red flushed face as if drunk, and because of repeated downpour into the groin, there is difficult urination, and periodically recurring muddledness.

Analysis:

- The original qì of the kidney was already debilitated and *Xiǎo Qīng Lóng Tāng* was erroneously administered.
- This leads to the stirring and surging of conception vessel fire, with vacuous qì surging upwards and vacuous yáng straying outwards.
- Therefore, the formula uses *guì zhī* and *fú líng* to absorb the upward surging qì.
- When *wǔ wèi zǐ* is combined with these other medicinals, the floating and straying of yáng can be restrained.

桂苓五味甘草去桂加薑辛湯
Guì Líng Wǔ Wèi Gān Cǎo Qù Guì Jiā Jiāng Xīn Tāng

fú líng	茯苓	12g
gān cǎo	甘草	9g
gān jiāng	乾薑	9g
xì xīn	細辛	9g
wǔ wèi zǐ	五味子	100ml

Indications: A treatment following the ingestion of the previous formula, which has lowered the surging qì, but now there is coughing and chest fullness.

Analysis:

- The strength of *guì zhī* and *fú líng* was able to lower the surging qì.
- Now, cold rheum is soaking the lungs resulting in coughing.
- Phlegm-rheum stored in the chest results in fullness.
- The great heat and acridity of *gān jiāng* and *xì xīn* must be used in order to discharge fullness from the chest and stop coughing.
- *Guì zhī* is only able to eliminate congealed and stagnant cold from the yáng aspect, and is unable to expel deep and hidden cold from the viscera and bowels, therefore it is removed from this formula.

苓甘五味薑辛半夏湯
Líng Gān Wǔ Wèi Jiāng Xīn Bàn Xià Tāng

fú líng	茯苓	12g
gān cǎo	甘草	9g
xì xīn	細辛	9g
gān jiāng	乾薑	9g
bàn xià	半夏	100ml
wǔ wèi zǐ	五味子	100ml

Indications: A treatment following the ingestion of the previous formula *Guì Líng Wǔ Wèi Gān Cǎo Qù Guì Jiā Jiāng Xīn Tāng*, which has stopped the coughing and chest fullness, but thirst and surging qì have returned.

Analysis:

- This formula is *Guì Líng Wǔ Wèi Gān Cǎo Qù Guì Jiā Jiāng Xīn Tāng* with the addition of *bàn xià.*
- Coughing and fullness have been eliminated, but thirst and surging qì have returned, as the heat of *xì xīn* and *gān jiāng* have caused agitation.
- If thirst on the contrary stops, this is due to surplus of rheum, and this restrains the dryness.
- When rheum is eliminated there is thirst, and when rheum returns, there is an absence of thirst with dizziness and vomiting.
- Therefore, use *bàn xià* to downbear counterflow, alleviate the dizziness, and vomiting.
- Other editions remove the *gān cǎo* out of fear that its sweetness will provoke vomiting.

苓甘五味薑辛半夏杏仁湯
Líng Gān Wǔ Wèi Jiāng Xīn Bàn Xià Xìng Rén Tāng

fú líng	茯苓	12g
gān cǎo	甘草	9g
gān jiāng	乾薑	9g
xì xīn	細辛	9g
wǔ wèi zǐ	五味子	100ml
bàn xià	半夏	100ml
xìng rén	杏仁	100ml

Indications: A treatment following the ingestion of the previous formula *Líng Gān Wǔ Wèi Jiāng Xīn Bàn Xià Tāng* where water was eliminated and vomiting has stopped, and now the patient has generalized swelling.

Analysis:

- Form and qì are ruled by the lungs.
- The lungs rule the skin and body hair, and are the officials in charge of the management and regulation of qì and water.
- Generalized swelling is the result of lung qì failing to move, and with congealing of qì there is lack of free flow.
- By adding *xìng rén*, we are able to drain due to its bitterness and open with its acridity, thereby freeing lung qì internally, and dissipating water qì in the exterior.
- *Má huáng* is not used because if yáng qì is diffused in vacuous patients, fluids could be seriously damaged.

苓甘五味薑辛夏杏大黄湯
Líng Gān Wǔ Wèi Jiāng Xīn Xià Xìng Dà Huáng Tāng

fú líng	茯苓	12g
gān cǎo	甘草	9g
gān jiāng	乾薑	9g
xì xīn	細辛	9g
wǔ wèi zǐ	五味子	100ml
bàn xià	半夏	100ml
xìng rén	杏仁	100ml
dà huáng	大黃	9g

Indications: Treats stomach heat surging upward and fuming the face manifesting with facial flushing as if drunk.

Analysis:

- Surging qì ascending counterflow with flushing as if drunk, and stomach heat surging upwards with facial flushing as if drunk, are not the same.
- The former is caused by yáng vacuity within yīn in the lower burner; while the latter of this pattern is the result of lung qì failing to move. When lung qì stagnates in the exterior, it causes generalized swelling; when lung qì stagnates in the interior, it causes stomach heat.
- *Xìng rén* disinhibits qì in the chest, and *dà huáng* discharges heat in the stomach, bringing forth resolution of the condition.

小半夏加茯苓湯
Xiǎo Bàn Xià Jiā Fú Líng Tāng

bàn xià	半夏	200ml
shēng jiāng	生薑	24g
fú líng	茯苓	9g

See above.

腎氣丸
Shèn Qì Wán

See above.

五苓散
Wǔ Líng Sǎn

See above.

文蛤散
Wén Gé Sǎn

wén gé	文蛤	15g

Indications: Treats cold damage tàiyáng disease with millet papules on the skin, a desire to drink water with an absence of actual thirst, or thirst with an incessant desire to drink water.

Analysis:

- Millet papules on the skin with an absence of actual thirst are the result of cold water soaking the lungs. The cold water gushes into the exterior, obstructing the upper burner, and covers the heat preventing it from being eliminated.
- *Wén gé* enters the lung, downbears lung qì, eliminates damp-heat, and disinhibits urination.
- Here a strategy of using a shell to treat the shell[3] is utilized.
- Thirst with incessant drinking of water has three possible causes: obstruction and depression of water-damp in the upper burner; dryness heat in the center that sets fire to the upper burner; dryness of the spleen and stomach with failure to engender fluids and quench thirst.
- Therefore, *wén gé's* salty flavor and cold nature is able to nourish yīn, moisten dryness, and eliminate heat qì by descending outwards through urination. Thus wén gé eliminates dry heat, promotes the growth of yīn, and alleviates thirst.

栝蔞瞿麥丸
Guā Lóu Qú Mài Wán

shǔ yù	薯蕷	9g
fú líng	茯苓	9g
guā lóu gēn	栝蔞根	6g
fù zǐ	附子	1 pc
qú mài	瞿麥	3g

Indications: Treats inhibited urination, thirst and cold in the abdomen.

Analysis:

- Within the formula *guā lóu gén* clears heat in the upper burner.
- *Fú líng* and *shǔ yù* supplements the earth of the central burner.

3. I.e. the exterior.

- *Fù zǐ* supplements the fire of the lower burner.
- *Qú mài* moves and frees the waterways, clears [the] source [of the urination] and simultaneously manages its flow.

蒲灰散
Pú Huī Sǎn

pú huī	蒲灰	½ part
huá shí	滑石	3 parts

Indications: Treats inhibited urination, and adverse skin water.

Analysis:
- When urination is inhibited, it should be expelled and discharged, otherwise water runs counterflow into the interstices of the flesh, resulting in skin water.
- The formula uses *pú huī* to dissipate water from the skin, and *huá shí* to free obstructed urination. As a result, a profound effect is achieved.

滑石白魚散
Huá Shí Bái Yú Sǎn

huá shí	滑石	2 parts
luàn fà	亂發	2 parts
bái yú	白魚	2 parts

Indications: Treats thirst, inhibited urination, distention, and pain in the lower abdomen, as a result of static blood.

Analysis:
- *Bái yú* opens the stomach, descends qì, eliminates both water qì and the superabundance of blood, and treats a shifted bladder with urinary stoppage.
- In combination with *huá shí,* they enrich yīn, boost qì, and disinhibit urination.

茯苓戎鹽湯
Fú Líng Róng Yán Tāng

fú líng	茯苓	24g
bái zhú	白朮	6g
róng yán	戎鹽	1 pc

Indications: Treats desiccation and blood stasis in the bladder with inhibited urination.

Analysis:
- This formula is *Wǔ Líng Sǎn* with *zhū líng, zé xié* and *guì zhī* removed and *róng yán* added.
- It is a formula that enters the kidneys and eliminates yīn fire.
- *Róng yán* is salty, cold and enters the stomach. Because of its nature of moist precipitation, *róng yán* is able to fulfill its duty in the function of percolating and disinhibiting, thereby expelling water-dampness from the yīn aspect.

白虎加人參湯
Bái Hǔ Jiā Rén Shēn Tāng[4]

zhī mǔ	知母	18g
shí gāo	石膏	48g
gān cǎo	甘草	6g
jīng mǐ	粳米	120ml
rén shēn	人參	9g

豬苓湯
Zhū Líng Tāng

zhū líng	豬苓	3g
fú líng	茯苓	3g
ē jiāo	阿膠	3g
huá shí	滑石	3g
zé xiè	澤瀉	3g

Indications: Treats yángmíng disease with a floating pulse, heat effusion, and thirst with a desire to drink water. Also treats shàoyīn disease where there is diarrhea for six or seven days, cough, retching, thirst, heart vexation, and inability to sleep.

Analysis:

- Zhòngjǐng created *Zhū Líng Tāng* to move water and heat in both the yángmíng and shàoyīn channels.
- However, its purpose is to boost yīn and not to specifically disinhibit water.
- Now, in a cold damage exterior vacuity pattern, one must avoid exhaustion of yáng. This is the same as with interior heat, where one must consider exhaustion of yīn. When there is exhaustion of yīn, it is the yīn of the kidneys, which has been exhausted along with the fluids of the stomach domain.
- Therefore, with a yīn vacuity person, not only are the bowels unable to move easily, but the urination also fails to freely move.
- If one excessively percolates and disinhibits in a yīn vacuity pattern, then fluids will be further consumed and exhausted.
- In the formula, *ē jiāo's* nature is to moisten, and it can therefore nourish the yīn and enrich dryness.
- The nature of *huá shí* is to lubricate, eliminate heat, and disinhibit water.
- The above functions are assisted by the percolating and draining of *fú líng* and *zhū líng*. Both of these medicinals dredge turbid heat and prevent it from settling, and thus obstructing and stagnating. In addition, they also moisten true yīn and prevent desiccation and dryness.
- Thus, this is an excellent formula to disinhibit water, and does not damage yīn.
- In order to disinhibit water in tàiyáng, use *Wǔ Líng Sǎn*. As tàiyáng is the office in charge of cold water, *guì zhī* is therefore used to warm the kidneys in order to move water.
- In yángmíng and shàoyīn disease use *Zhū Líng Tāng* as both channels are related to the fluids.
- The unique characteristic of *Zhū Líng Tāng* is the use of *ē jiāo* and *huá shí* to moisten, as they can nourish the formless and move that which has form.
- Although both *Wǔ Líng Sǎn* and *Zhū Líng Tāng* disinhibit water, they are differentiated by cold and heat, and only one who is clearly aware of these facts will be skilled in their use.

4. Refer to page 260 in Volume 1.

越婢加朮湯
Yuè Bì Jiā Zhú Tāng

má huáng	麻黃	18g
shí gāo	石膏	24g
shēng jiāng	生薑	6g
gān cǎo	甘草	9g
bái zhú	白朮	12g
dà zǎo	大棗	15 pcs

Indications: Water in the interior with yellow discoloration, swelling all over the body, face, and eyes, a sunken pulse, and inhibited urination. Also treats extreme heat in the interior with openness of the interstices and severe sweating, as well as pestilential wind qì with weakness in the lower burner and feet.

Analysis:

- *Yuè Bì Tāng* can disperse generalized swelling and also dissipate internally smoldering heat.
- *Bái zhú* is able to support the spleen and thereby control water. Hence, it can also secure the interstices and check sweating.
- However, if there is discharging of great sweat, it is appropriate to reduce the *má huáng*.
- For a more detailed description, refer to *Yùe Bì Tāng*.

防己黃芪湯
Fáng Jǐ Huáng Qí Tāng

fáng jǐ	防己	3g
gān cǎo	甘草	1.5g
bái zhú	白朮	2.25g
huáng qí	黃芪	3.75g

Indications: Wind-damp and wind-water, with vexing pain in the joints, a floating pulse, heavy body, and sweating with aversion to wind.

Analysis:

- Aversion to wind is due to wind damaging the interstices. Generalized heaviness is due to dampness damaging the channels and network vessels. The floating pulse is due to an exterior disease.
- Why would one not use *guì zhī* or *má huáng* to effuse the exterior and eliminate wind, but instead use *fáng jǐ* and *huáng qí* to supplement vacuity and move water? This is because the sweating here is due to vacuity of the interstices, and the generalized heaviness is the result of an earth vacuity with the prevalence of dampness.
- *Huáng qí* penetrates the exterior and fills up emptiness.
- *Dà zǎo, gān cǎo,* and *bái zhú* supplement earth and overcome dampness.
- *Shēng jiāng* drives out wind with its acridity and moves water with its warmth.
- *Fáng jǐ* penetrates everywhere, thereby leading the other medicinals to circulate throughout the entire body, freeing the outside and reaching the inside.

越婢湯
Yuè Bì Tāng

má huáng	麻黃	18g
shí gāo	石膏	24g
shēng jiāng	生薑	9g
gān cǎo	甘草	6g
dà zǎo	大棗	12 pcs

Indications: Treats wind-water with an aversion to wind, generalized swelling, a floating pulse, an absence of thirst, periodic spontaneous sweating, and an absence of great heat.

Analysis:

- This is a major formula used to treat water swelling.
- Water swelling is typically caused by lung qì failing to disseminate, and weak spleen qì.
- When the lungs are unable to move water, and the spleen is unable to stop water, this results in the congestion and stagnation of water in the channels and network vessels with swelling.
- In the formula *má huáng* courses the lung in order to move water in the three yáng channels and network vessels.
- *Shí gāo* is acrid and cool. *Shēng jiāng* is acrid and warm. Together they move both the hand and foot yángmíng channels and network vessels in order to reduce swelling in the flesh.
- *Dà zǎo* and *gān cǎo* are used to secure the qì of the spleen and stomach in the central burner.
- When there is aversion to wind *fù zǐ* is added, and this treats evil in the three yīn channels and network vessels.
- When there is wind-water *bái zhú* is added in order to support the earth and restrain water.

防己茯苓湯
Fáng Jǐ Fú Líng Tāng

fáng jǐ	防己	9g
huáng qí	黃芪	9g
guì zhī	桂枝	9g
fú líng	茯苓	18g
gān cǎo	甘草	6g

Indications: Treats skin water disease with swelling of the four extremities.

Analysis:

- This formula contains the same medicinals as *Fáng Jǐ Huáng Qí Tāng*, but with *bái zhú* removed, and *guì zhī*, and *fú líng* added.
- The dampness of wind-water is in the channels and network vessels close to the interior, and the dampness of skin water is in the skin close to the exterior.
- Therefore, we only need *fú líng* to assist *guì zhī* in percolating dampness throughout the entire body, and there is no need to use *bái zhú* to dry the center qì.
- Neither *shēng jiāng* or *dà zǎo* are used, as dampness is not in the construction or defense of the upper burner, and does not need to be diffused.

越婢加朮湯
Yuè Bì Jiā Zhú Tāng

See above.

甘草麻黄湯
Gān Cǎo Má Huáng Tāng

gān cǎo	甘草	6g
má huáng	麻黄	12g

Indications: Treats interior water diseases.

Analysis:
- This formula uses *má huáng*, as it is the quickest medicinal to promote sweat.
- Xū Língtāi said that *má huáng* is one without qì, flavor, or an affinity to a specific channel, and indeed reaches all channels.
- Since *má huáng* comes from empty space, all substantial qì and blood would be unable to handle it.

麻黄附子湯
Má Huáng Fù Zǐ Tāng

má huáng	麻黄	9g
gān cǎo	甘草	6g
fù zǐ	附子	1 pc

Indications: Treats shàoyīn disease with a deep pulse and heat effusion. Also, treats water swelling with a deep pulse.

Analysis:
- When cold damage reaches shàoyīn, it has already entered the deepest portion of the lower burner.
- Therefore, although the formula contains *má huáng* to effuse evil in the three yáng channels, without the use of *fù zǐ's* swift freeing of the three yīn channels and network vessels, one will most certainly be unable to thrust out interior disease evil into the exterior.
- Generalized water swelling is due to the kidney viscus being unable to expel and discharge.
- The kidneys belong to shàoyīn, and *fù zǐ* is the main medicinal used to free the shàoyīn channels and network vessels; therefore it is quite suitable here.
- Since *má huáng* and *fù zǐ* are both fierce and harsh medicinals, *gān cǎo* is used to moderate and harmonize them, and this is the method used to restrain in this formula.

杏子湯
Xìng Zǐ Tāng

Please refer to the formula on page 82 for a detailed discussion regarding the discrepancies in *Xìng Zǐ Tāng's* ingredients.

Indications: Treats cold damage with an absence of sweating and panting, sweating with panting, or panting following precipitation. Also treats a wind-warmth exterior repletion pattern with an absence of sweating, spontaneous sweating, headache, generalized body pain, generalized heaviness, copious sleeping, snoring, difficult speech, vexing thirst, aversion to heat, and a floating pulse.

Analysis:
- This formula treats a pattern of heat in the lung domain.
- It uses *xìng rén* to disinhibit lung qì in order to settle panting.
- *Má huáng* resolves the fleshy exterior in order to dissipate heat, and at the same time *shí gāo* is added to clear heat.

- *Gān cǎo* is used to harmonize.
- Therefore, in the absence of sweating with a closed exterior, one can give *má huáng* to obtain a sweat.
- When there is internal heat with spontaneous sweating, one can give *shí gāo* to stop sweating.
- After cold damage has transformed into heat, the evil has still not departed from the lung, and so this formula can be given to clear and resolve it.
- In all patterns of wind-warmth with latent evil, this evil has accumulated and is oppressed in the lungs, and therefore this formula can be given in order to course and dissipate it.
- This really is an excellent formula for treating diseases with heat in the upper burner.
- However, if the disease is not in the lungs, or in patterns where an absence of heat is observed, it is not suitable to give this formula.
- Therefore, a floating pulse is the standard sign warranting its use, and is contraindicated with aversion to cold and an absence of thirst.

蒲灰散
Pú Huī Sǎn

See above.

黄芪芍藥桂枝苦酒湯
Huáng Qí Sháo Yào Guì Zhī Kǔ Jiǔ Tāng

huáng qí	黄芪	15g
sháo yào	芍藥	9g
guì zhī	桂枝	9g

Indications: Treats yellow sweat disease, with generalized swelling, heat effusion, sweating with thirst, and a deep pulse.

Analysis:

- This disease arises when one takes a bath while sweating, and water enters through the pores.
- The water becomes depressed, steams, and turns into heat. Dampness and heat will interact, brew and bind in the pores and fail to resolve, and thus result in yellow sweat disease.
- The formula uses *guì zhī* to move yáng.
- *Sháo yào* boosts yīn.
- The qì and flavor of *huáng qí* is light and clear with the outer skin being the most rich, therefore, it can reach the skin quite swiftly.
- This decoction is boiled with vinegar, as the sour taste of the vinegar can directly assist in stopping sweating.

桂枝加黄芪湯
Guì Zhī Jiā Huáng Qí Tāng

guì zhī	桂枝	9g
sháo yào	芍藥	9g
shēng jiāng	生薑	9g
gān cǎo	甘草	6g
huáng qí	黄芪	6g
dà zǎo	大棗	12 pcs

Indications: Treats yellow sweat disease and jaundice with a floating pulse.

Analysis:

- In yellow sweat with a floating pulse, the disease is in the fleshy exterior.
- Therefore, *Guì Zhī Tāng* is used to harmonize the construction and defense by resolving the flesh and effusing the exterior.
- *Huáng qí* is good at penetrating the skin to effuse sweat and abate yellowing.
- It is combined with acrid *shēng jiāng* and *guì zhī*, so the depressed dampness and heat in the fleshy exterior does not become troublesome and can be eliminated.

桂甘薑棗麻辛附子湯
Guì Gān Jiāng Zǎo Má Xīn Fù Zǐ Tāng

guì zhī	桂枝	9g
shēng jiāng	生薑	9g
xì xīn	細辛	6g
gān cǎo	甘草	6g
má huáng	麻黄	6g
fù zǐ	附子	1 pc
dà zǎo	大棗	12 pcs

The alternate name of this formula is *Guì Zhī Qù Sháo Yào Jiā Má Xīn Fù Zǐ Tāng*.

Indications: A treatment for qì aspect disease with hardness below the heart the size of a platter with edges that resemble an overturned cup.

Analysis:

- This pattern belongs to a heart and kidney interaction disease, where the upper is unable to descend, and the lower is unable to ascend.
- After an extended period of time, it becomes hard to break like iron and stone.
- The formula uses *má huáng*, *guì zhī*, and *shēng jiāng* in order to attack the upper.
- *Fù zǐ*, and *xì xīn* are used to attack the lower.
- *Gān cǎo* and *dà zǎo* are used to supplement the central burner in order to transport qì.
- Once there is interaction between the qì of the upper and lower, the disease can be cured.
- It is said that once the great qì shifts, the bind will immediately dissipate.
- *Sháo yào* is removed to avoid its sour contracting effect.

枳朮湯
Zhǐ Zhú Tāng

zhǐ shí	枳實	7 pcs
bái zhú	白朮	6g

Indications: Treats hardness below the heart, which is the size of a platter, with edges that resemble an overturned cup. This is due to water-rheum. Also treats postpartum puffy swelling edema.

Analysis:

- The area below the heart, is the region of the upper stomach duct.
- Binding and hardness in the upper stomach duct with edges that resemble an overturned cup, which fluctuates in size sometimes big and sometimes small, is due to water qì, and is not the result of food stagnation.
- The coldness of *zhǐ shí* is used in order to break bound qì.

- The warmth of *bái zhú* is used in order to eliminate water-dampness.
- When three doses are taken warm, the abdomen softens and the bind opens.
- As a result the hardness is eliminated.
- Lǐ Gǎo's[5] method when applying this formula was to double the *bái zhú*, as supplementation was his main objective.
- However, the sovereign of this formula is *zhǐ shí*, as drainage is the main objective of the formula.
- Thus, in differentiating these two treatment styles: one moderates, while the other treats urgently; and one supplements, while the other drains. These usages are thus quite different, and is only determined by the dosage of the medicinals.

《外臺》防己黃芪湯
Wài Tái Fáng Jǐ Huáng Qí Tāng

See above.

茵陳蒿湯
Yīn Chén Hāo Tāng

yīn chén hāo	茵陳蒿	18g
zhī zǐ	梔子	14 pcs
dà huáng	大黃	6g

Indications: Treats yángmíng disease with heat effusion, sweating only from the head, and not from the body, inhibited urination, and thirst with intake of fluids. This indicates stasis heat in the interior, and as a result, there will be generalized yellowing. This formula also treats cold damage, which has lasted for seven or eight days with generalized yellowing the color of a tangerine, inhibited urination, and mild abdominal fullness.

Analysis:

- The yellowing occurs in both tàiyáng and yángmìng patterns.
- However, when there is only sweating from the head and not from the body, then heat is unable to move outwards. When the urination is inhibited, heat is unable to drain downwards. This results in stasis heat in the interior. However, even amongst the interior patterns, there are differences.
- The flesh is the interior of tàiyáng and is from where sweat should emit. Thus, *Má Huáng Lián Qiào Chì Xiǎo Dòu Tāng* is the formula used to cool and dissipate.
- The heart and chest are the interior of tàiyáng and yángmíng, and are dominated by cold.
- *Zhī Zǐ Bǎi Pí Tāng* is a method used to clear fire.
- The intestines and stomach are the interior of yángmíng, and should be drained from the interior. Therefore, immediately use this formula, as it expels filth.
- As the stalks of *yīn chén* do not wither and die in the winter, they receive the qì of great cold, and can therefore eliminate evil heat that has settled and bound.
- *Zhī zǐ* is used to free the source of water.
- *Dà huáng* eliminates intestinal repletion.

5. Lǐ Dōngyuán 李東垣, also known as Lǐ Gǎo 李杲, was one of the "Four Masters of the *Jīn-Yuán* period" 金元四大家, the author of the *Pí Wèi Lùn* 《脾胃論》(Treatise on the Spleen and Stomach), and the founder of the Supplementing-Earth School (*bǔ tǔ pài* 補土派). He lived from 1180–1251.

- As a result both interior and exterior static heat are eliminated through urination, abdominal fullness is reduced, and there is no damage to the stomach and intestines.
- This is a sacred formula used to disinhibit yángmíng water.
- As for inhibited urination and slight abdominal fullness, one can also use this formula.
- *Yīn chén* pushes out the old to make room for the new, and is assisted by *zhī zǐ*, which facilitates downward movement.
- In this case, *hòu pò* and *zhǐ shí* are not used to coordinate the qì downwards nor is *máng xiāo* used to harshly disinhibit.
- By using *dà huáng* to moisten the stomach the stools are thereby not moved all at once, and only then will the abiding accumulations in the stomach be reduced.
- In this case the yellowing jaundice is expelled through urination.

硝石礬石散
Xiāo Shí Fán Shí Sǎn

xiāo shí	硝石	equal parts
fán shí	礬石	equal parts

Indications: Treats sexual taxation jaundice and black jaundice.

Analysis:

- *Xiāo shí* can dissipate vacuous depressed heat causing [it to be] lightly shed from the body, while its coldness will not damage the spleen.
- *Fán shí* is able to eliminate water, so water evil is not able to invade wherever *fán shí* goes, and like paper *fán shí* does not allow for seepage of water.
- These medicinals are taken mixed with barley gruel, which boosts earth in order to overcome water. When the medicinals are combined, they can dissipate depressed heat, and resolve kidney toxicity.
- Here, there are no methods that involve qì, blood, yīn, yáng, sweating, precipitating, supplementing or draining in the least. However, it is still an excellent formula.

梔子大黃湯
Zhī Zǐ Dà Huáng Tāng

zhī zǐ	梔子	14 pcs
dà huáng	大黃	6g
zhǐ shí	枳實	5 pcs
chǐ	豉	200ml

Indications: Treats liquor jaundice with anguish in the heart, or heat pain.

Analysis:

- This formula is used due to damage of the yīn aspect from liquor.
- Therefore, drying medicinals are contraindicated in order to avoid consuming liquids, as are percolating medicinals, which can exhaust humors.
- The upper and the lower are separately dispersed, and heat qì is smoothly coordinated downwards. As a result, the disease can be resolved.

桂枝加黃芪湯
Guì Zhī Jiā Huáng Qí Tāng

guì zhī	桂枝	9g
sháo yào	芍藥	9g
shēng jiāng	生薑	9g
dà zǎo	大棗	12 pcs
gān cǎo	甘草	6g
huáng qí	黃芪	6g

See above.

豬膏發煎
Zhū Gāo Fā Jiān

zhū gāo	豬膏	24g
luàn fà	亂發	3 pcs

Indications: Treats all jaundice diseases, sexual taxation jaundice, downward drainage of stomach qì in women, and vaginal flatulence characterized by an incessant loud sound.

Analysis:

- *Zhū gāo* rules the moistening of dryness.
- *Luàn fà* rules the freeing of urination.
- In the *Shén Nóng Běn Cǎo Jīng* there is a very ingenious and exemplary sentence that states: hair is the surplus of blood, whereby water essence is received by the heart, and is transformed into blood.
- Nowadays, this formula is taken processed, which is still capable of entering the yīn organs. It assists water essence to ascend and be received by the spirit of the heart, in order to be transformed into blood.

茵陳五苓散
Yīn Chén Wǔ Líng Sǎn

yīn chén	茵陳	10 parts
wǔ líng sǎn	五苓散	5 parts

Indications: Treats jaundice.

Analysis:

- Jaundice is due to dampness, heat stasis, and depression steaming upwards, thus causing yellowing.
- Unless *yīn chén hāo* is used to push out the old to make room for the new, one cannot eliminate heat and abate jaundice.
- In addition, unless *Wǔ Líng Sǎn* is used to shift and transport water, one cannot promote sweating and move water.
- By using these two together, both the interior and exterior are resolved.

大黃硝石湯
Dà Huáng Xiāo Shí Tāng

dà huáng	大黃	12g
huáng bǎi	黃柏	12g
xiāo shí	硝石	12g
zhī zǐ	梔子	15 pcs

Indications: Treats jaundice with abdominal fullness, inhibited and red urination, and spontaneous sweating.

Analysis:

- In this pattern the exterior is in harmony and there is heat in the interior.
- *Dà huáng* is used to eliminate fullness and repletion.

- *Xiāo shí* leads heat qì downwards through the stool and urine.

小半夏湯
Xiǎo Bàn Xià Tāng

bàn xià	半夏	200ml
shēng jiāng	生薑	24g

See above.

小柴胡湯
Xiǎo Chái Hú Tāng

chái hú	柴胡	24g
huáng qín	黃芩	9g
rén shēn	人參	9g
gān cǎo	甘草	6g
bàn xià	半夏	24g
shēng jiāng	生薑	9g
dà zǎo	大棗	12 pcs

Indications: Treats cold damage with aversion to wind, alternating fever and chills, bitter fullness in the chest and rib-sides, taciturnity with a lack of desire to eat, heart vexation with a desire to vomit, bitter taste in the mouth, deafness, and a wiry rapid pulse. There may also be vexation in the chest with no retching, thirst or an absence of thirst, slight heat in the body, possible abdominal pain, possible hard glomus in the rib-sides, possible palpitations below the heart, inhibited urination, and possible cough, all of which belong to a shàoyáng channel half-exterior half-interior pattern. In treatment it is appropriate to harmonize and resolve.

Analysis:

- This is the main formula used to harmonize and resolve a half-exterior half-interior shàoyáng channel pattern.
- The shàoyáng channel and network vessels follow the rib-sides and ascend to the space between the abdomen and the back. This is the common boundary between yīn and yáng, and is the location where evil transmits.
- When evil is in the exterior and is about to enter the interior, but interior qì resists it, then there is alternating fever and chills with bitter fullness in the chest and rib-sides.
- When there is a struggle between the right qì and evil, this results in a clouded spirit and taciturnity.
- When wood invades earth there is a lack of desire to eat and retching.
- When evil heat distresses the interior there is heart vexation.
- When gallbladder fire spills upwards there is a bitter taste in the mouth.
- When there is heat in the shàoyáng channel this results in deafness.
- The formula uses *chái hú* to course and dissipate the shàoyáng channel and network vessel in order to outthrust evil from the half-exterior half-interior.
- *Bàn xià* harmonizes the stomach.
- *Huáng qín* clears heat in the half-interior preventing the inward penetration of evil.
- *Rén shēn* supplements vacuity and assists in generating and effusing qì.
- *Gān cǎo* assists *chái hú* and *huáng qín* in harmonizing the interior and exterior.
- *Shēng jiāng* and *dà zǎo* assist *rén shēn* and *bàn xià* in the freeing of the construction and defense, and in alleviating cold and heat.

- All of the medicinals are mutually enhancing making this an excellent formula.
- If there is vexation in the chest and no retching, this means there is only heat in the stomach, which has not yet become disharmonized. Use *guā lóu* to flush out the heat, and there is no need to use *rén shēn* and *bàn xià* to harmonize the stomach.
- When there is abdominal pain due to shàoyáng wind-wood invading spleen earth, it is appropriate to remove bitter cold *huáng qín* and add *sháo yào* in order to drain wood.
- If there is rib-side glomus as a result of extreme liver evil, then it is appropriate to remove sticky *dà zǎo*, and add *mǔ lì* in order to emolliate the liver.
- When there is heart palpitations and inhibited urination due to water evil failing to discharge outwards, which thus internally invades the heart, then remove *huáng qín* and add *fú líng* in order to percolate water.
- If there is an absence of thirst with slight heat in the exterior due to the incomplete elimination of evils, remove sticky *rén shēn*, and add *guì zhī* in order to resolve the exterior.
- When there is cough due to evil in the lungs, remove the enriching and supplementing *rén shēn* and *dà zǎo*, and add *wǔ wèi zǐ* and *gān jiāng* to warm and dissipate.
- Now if there are only wind-cold true malaria evils in the shàoyáng and construction yīn is not depleted, then this formula can be used.
- If there is malaria due to warm disease or summer-heat disease with breathing from the mouth and nose, this is due to deep-lying heat in the lungs and stomach. If the formula is also freely used, then heat evil will increase with the use of *chái hú*. The use of *rén shēn* and *gān cǎo* will also cause heat in the lungs and stomach to increase and stagnate. This in turn causes the lodging of yīn and yáng evils, and thus they are not effectively treated.

小建中湯
Xiǎo Jiàn Zhōng Tāng

guì zhī	桂枝	9g
gān cǎo	甘草	6g
dà zǎo	大棗	12 pcs
sháo yào	芍藥	18g
shēng jiāng	生薑	9g
jiāo yí	膠飴	200ml

Indications: Unresolved cold damage in the exterior, with a rough yáng pulse and a wiry yīn pulse, vexation and palpitations in the heart, with tension and pain in the abdomen. This treats vacuity taxation with abdominal urgency, palpitations, nosebleed, and abdominal pain. It also treats seminal loss during dreaming, soreness in the four extremities, vexing heat in the hands and feet, as well as dry throat and mouth.

Analysis:

- This formula is *Guì Zhī Tāng* with double the amount of *sháo yào*, and the addition of malt sugar.
- Palpitations means yáng vacuity; vexation means yīn vacuity. Cold qì entering the yáng network vessels makes the yáng pulse rough; entering the yīn network vessels makes the yīn pulse wiry.
- Insufficiency in the construction and defense means vacuity in the exterior.

- Wind entering earth signifies tension in the interior.
- Even though the center is vacuous, the exterior is not yet harmonized. Therefore do not supplement strongly yet!
- With its bitterness and sourness, the sovereign *sháo yào* boosts yīn, and is able to drain wood from within earth.
- The warmth of the ministers' malt sugar and *gān cǎo* supplements the spleen and nourishes the stomach.
- The acrid heat of *guì zhī* is used to support yáng and remove cold water.
- The acrid warmth of the envoys *shēng jiāng* and *dà zǎo* are able to dissipate yáng qì.
- Take the formula warm to cause sweating.
- The emphasis of the formula is on treating the vacuity in the center, not the cold damage in the exterior.
- Because of the sweetness, this formula is contraindicated in patients suffering from retching and also for alcoholics.

瓜蒂散
Guā Dì Sǎn

guā dì	瓜蒂	1 part
chì xiǎo dòu	赤小豆	1 part

Indications: Treats a floating *cùn* pulse with glomus in the chest, and abiding food in the upper stomach duct.

Analysis:
- Main formula for inducing vomiting.
- For conditions caused by cold, heat, damp turbidity, and phlegm-rheum brewing and binding in the chest.
- For conditions where treatment by promoting sweating or precipitation is ineffective.
- Formula uses sour and bitter emetics to free the upper burner and allow yáng qì to return.
- The formula uses the extreme bitterness of *guā dì* and the sour, descending nature of *chì xiǎo dòu*, to mutually benefit each other. Together these two medicinals eliminate repletion evil from the chest and stomach.
- Taking this together with *xiāng chǐ* gruel to protect stomach qì, can increase the efficacy of the formula.
- If no vomiting results, increase the dosage very slowly. As soon as vomiting occurs, stop immediately to prevent damage to the original qì of the stomach.

《千金》麻黄醇酒湯
Qiān Jīn Má Huáng Chún Jiǔ Tāng

má huáng	麻黄	9g
chún jiǔ	醇酒	1000ml

Indications: Treats jaundice.

Analysis:
- *Má huáng* is light, clear, and penetrates the exterior. It is a qì aspect medicinal, which rules exterior repletion patterns with an absence of sweating.
- Jaundice is considered to be linked to dampness and heat evils, and for this reason *Má Huáng Chún Jiǔ Tāng* is used.
- Jaundice resides in the fleshy exterior between the nutritive and defense.

- Without *má huáng* one would be unable to move the fleshy exterior, and unless clear liquor is used, one would be unable to free the nutritive and defense.
- Therefore, *má huáng* is boiled in clear liquor in order to assist in its function of promoting sweat. When sweat flows, then the nutritive and defense is free, and one knows that the evil, which is hidden internally, is resolved through the exterior.
- *Mǔ lì's* water nature restrains fire evil.
- *Lóng gǔ's* heavy nature settles floating and straying.
- *Gān cǎo, dà zǎo,* and *shēng jiāng* all support and assist the essence of water and grains of the central burner.
- *Shào yào* is removed due to its bitter flavor and balanced nature. It would only be appropriate to use in the absence of yáng collapse.

桂枝去芍藥加蜀漆牡蠣龍骨救逆湯
Guì Zhī Qù Sháo Yào Jiā Shǔ Qī Mǔ Lì Lóng Gǔ Jiù Nì Tāng

guì zhī	桂枝	9g
gān cǎo	甘草	6g
shēng jiāng	生薑	9g
dà zǎo	大棗	12 pcs
mǔ lì	牡蠣	15g
shǔ qī	蜀漆	9g
lóng gǔ	龍骨	12g

Indications: Treats cold damage with a floating pulse where fire treatment was used to force sweating causing yáng collapse and fright mania. There is also disquietude whether lying or standing up; this also treats fire evil.

Analysis:

- Tàiyáng and the sovereign fire are mutually connected.
- Here, there is yáng collapse of the sovereign heart.
- This is different than the collapse of yáng associated with shàoyīn sweating.
- Therefore, *guì zhī* is used to protect heart qì.
- *Shǔ qī* frees yáng and drains heat.

半夏麻黃丸
Bàn Xià Má Huáng Wán

bàn xià	半夏	equal parts
má huáng	麻黃	equal parts

Indications: Treats cold rheum stoppage and amassment with palpitations, and a floating, tight pulse.

Analysis:

- This formula uses *bàn xià* to eliminate rheum qì, and *má huáng* to effuse yáng qì.
- The ingenuity lies in the processing and administration of the pills, which function to moderately resolve the condition.
- The acrid and sweet flavor of *má huáng* is unable to diffuse liquid qì, and can only upbear yáng qì.
- In addition, the bitter and acrid flavor of *bàn xià* not only eliminates rheum qì, but also harmonizes and nourishes center qì.

柏葉湯
Bǎi Yè Tāng

bǎi yè	柏葉	9g
gān jiāng	乾薑	9g
ài	艾	3 handfuls

Indications: Treats incessant vomiting of blood.

Analysis:

- Incessant counterflow of blood must be blamed on effulgent fire.
- Therefore, *bǎi yè* is used to treat the effulgent qì.
- It is combined with acrid and warm *ài yè* and *gān jiāng*, which can dissipate binds, and prevent stagnation.
- Horse manure liquid is used in order to guide downwards.

黄土湯
Huáng Tǔ Tāng

gān cǎo	甘草	9g
gān dì huáng	乾地黄	9g
bái zhú	白朮	9g
fù zǐ	附子	9g
ē jiāo	阿膠	9g
huáng qín	黄芩	9g
zào zhōng huáng tǔ	竈中黄土	24g

Indications: Treats blood ejection, nosebleeds, and blood precipitation where bleeding follows the stools. This also treats menstrual flooding in women.

Analysis:

- Patterns of blood descent where there is first bleeding followed by stools, is related to damage of the spleen network vessels.
- When there is permeation of blood in the intestines, and stasis accumulation in the lower, the stools fail to move and blood descends first. In this case, Zhòngjǐng mainly used *Chì Xiǎo Dāng Guī Sǎn.*
- When there are first stools followed by bleeding, this is is related to the blood of the liver channel and diverging network vessel.
- When the spleen is vacuous, yáng sinks and generates dampness, then blood descends following the dampness. In this case, Zhòngjǐng mainly used *Huáng Tǔ Tāng,* which is warming, drying, and eliminates cold and dampness.
- The ministers' *shēng dì huáng, ē jiāo,* and *huáng qín* enter the liver and treat blood heat.
- The assistants' *bái zhú, gān cǎo,* and *fù zǐ* support the yáng and supplement the spleen in order to treat the vacuous root.
- In this formula, forty-eight grams of *chì shí zhī* can be used instead of *zào zhōng huáng tǔ.* Six grams of *páo jiāng* can be substituted for *fù zǐ,* but *páo fù zǐ* is even better.

赤小豆散
Chì Xiǎo Dòu Sǎn

chì xiǎo dòu	赤小豆	600ml
dāng guī	當歸	no quantity given

Indications: Treats fox-creeper disease and blood in the stools.

Analysis:

- For damp-heat invading the genitals.
- *Chì xiǎo dòu* removes dampness, clears heat, and resolves toxin, treating disease in the shàoyīn.
- *Dāng guī* leads heat down, nourishes blood, disperses depression, and treats disease in the juéyīn.
- Taking the powder by drinking it with fermented grain-water harmonizes stomach qì.
- When stomach qì and shàoyīn are in harmony, then fire and earth are united and virtuous.
- When earth and wood are obedient, juéyīn is in harmony.
- As a result the fox-creeper disease and blood in the stools spontaneously resolve.

瀉心湯
Xiè Xīn Tāng

dà huáng	大黄	6g
huáng lián	黄連	3g
huáng qín	黄芩	3g

Indications:
1) Treats insufficiency of heart qì with blood ejection, nosebleed, accumulation of heat in the heart, delirious speech, mania, and a desire to climb over walls and onto roofs.
2) Treats women with ejection of foamy drool that was inappropriately precipitated, which immediately manifests with glomus below the heart. One should treat the ejection of foamy drool first, and *Xiǎo Qīng Lóng Tāng* rules it. Once the ejection of foamy drool has stopped, then treat the glomus, and this decoction rules it.

Analysis:

- When fire evil is exuberant and distresses the blood, this leads to derangement of the channels with frenetic movement.
- Blood is the humor of the heart, and when damaged, fails to nourish the heart resulting in an insufficiency of the qì of heart yīn.
- Therefore, this is called insufficiency of the heart qì, and not insufficiency of the qì of heart yáng.
- Bitter and cold medicinals *huáng qín* and *huáng lián* enter the heart and clear fire in order to bank up heart qì.
- *Dà huáng* eliminates stasis and engenders the new.
- This is a method of treatment in which both supplementation and drainage are used.

吳茱萸湯
Wú Zhū Yú Tāng

wú zhū yú	吳茱萸	200ml
rén shēn	人參	9g
shēng jiāng	生薑	18g
dà zǎo	大棗	12 pcs

Indications: Treats cold damage retching and chest fullness. Possibly also with vexation, agitation, and a desire to die.

Analysis:
- The chest is the location of yáng, which is vast like the sky.
- When there is retching and chest fullness, yīn evil has occupied the position of yáng.
- Therefore, large doses of the majorly acrid and warm *shēng jiāng* and *wú zhū yú* are used in order to free yáng within the chest, and break the haze of qì.
- The assistants *rén shēn* and *dà zǎo*, one being yīn the other yáng, fortify spleen and stomach qì in order to settle the counterflow of ascending yīn, enabling the sunlight to illuminate everything, which results in the dispersion of concealed yīn.
- How then could there be any more trouble with dry retching, chest fullness, drool and spittle?

半夏瀉心湯
Bàn Xià Xiè Xīn Tāng

bàn xià	半夏	100ml
huáng qín	黃芩	9g
gān jiāng	乾薑	9g
rén shēn	人參	9g
huáng lián	黃連	3g
dà zǎo	大棗	12 pcs
gān cǎo	甘草	9g

Indications: Treats cold damage glomus below the heart and retching with intestinal rumbling.

Analysis:
- Glomus below the heart is the result of damp-heat depression and stagnation in the stomach, which upon rising results in retching.
- When it descends, there is intestinal rumbling.
- The sovereign of the formula is *bàn xià*, which harmonizes the stomach.
- *Gān jiāng's* acrid warmth serves to open the stomach.
- *Huáng qín* and *huáng lián* are bitter cold and discharge.
- *Rén shēn*, *gān cǎo*, and *dà zǎo* are sweet, warm, and supplementing.
- As a result, both dampness and stagnation are eliminated and the stomach qì is restored.
- The ingenuity lies in the boiling of the decoction again after removing the dregs, making it light and clear. This facilitates the easy movement and transformation of the stomach, transforms glomus, and downbears counterflow.

黃芩加半夏生薑湯
Huáng Qín Jiā Bàn Xià Shēng Jiāng Tāng

huáng qín	黃芩	9g
gān cǎo	甘草	6g
sháo yào	芍藥	6g
bàn xià	半夏	100ml
shēng jiāng	生薑	9g
dà zǎo	大棗	12 pcs

Indications: Treats tàiyáng and shàoyáng combination disease, with retching and an absence of diarrhea. Also treats dry retching and diarrhea.

Analysis:

- This is a major formula, which harmonizes the spleen and stomach.
- Retching is usually the result of a stomach disharmony.
- Retching with cough is due to the upward distressing of heat evil.
- Retching and diarrhea is the result of the lower distressing of heat evil.
- Dry retching with the arrival of bitter water[6] gastric secretions rising to the mouth is due to the exhaustion of stomach fluids.
- The formula uses *bàn xià* and *shēng jiāng* to harmonize the stomach, transform rheum, and eliminate fullness.
- *Sháo yào* drains liver and gallbladder fire and stops dry retching.
- *Huáng qín* clears fire from the lungs and intestines, as well as stops cough and diarrhea.
- *Gān cǎo* and *dà zǎo* are used to enrich the spleen and stomach, and alleviate the presence of bitter water.
- Thus, all patterns of center disharmony can be treated.
- Later generations of physicians have removed the *sháo yào* in order to concentrate the formula on the stomach.

小半夏湯
Xiǎo Bàn Xià Tāng

bàn xià	半夏	200ml
shēng jiāng	生薑	24g

See above.

豬苓散
Zhū Líng Sǎn

zhū líng	豬苓	equal parts of each
fú líng	茯苓	
bái zhú	白朮	

Indications: Treats vomiting with a desire for water.

四逆湯
Sì Nì Tāng

fù zǐ	附子	1 pc
gān jiāng	乾薑	4.5g
gān cǎo	甘草	6g

Indications: Treats shàoyīn disease with exterior heat and interior cold, clears grain diarrhea, hypertonicity of the limbs, reversal cold of the extremities, and a faint pulse which is verging on expiry.

6. Gastric secretions rising to the mouth.

Analysis:

- This is a drastic formula to warm the channels and rescue yáng.
- It rules the treatment of cold in both the center and exterior manifesting with reversal cold of the extermities.
- The sovereign is *zhì gān cǎo*, which is sweet and warm. On the exterior it warms the nutritive and defense, and in the interior it supplements the central burner.
- The ministers' *gān jiāng* and *fù zǐ* are acrid and warm. Together, they are able to ascend to the top of the head, penetrate the fleshy exterior, and free and move the twelve channels.
- When *gān jiāng* and *fù zǐ* are used combined with *gān cǎo* in the presence of water in the center, they are able to rouse kidney yáng, warm central cold, and warm the earth.
- When *gān cǎo* is used together with *gān jiāng* and *fù zǐ*, the joints are freed, the extremities are reached, yīn is expelled, and yáng is stemmed. Thus, kidney yáng is roused and yīn cold is dispersed, resulting in the opening of the vessels and the warming of the extremities.

- This is the reason why this is a major formula for treating the shàoyīn channel.
- Strong patients can use one large piece of *fù zǐ*, and nine grams of *gān jiāng*.
- This formula can be compared with *Má Huáng Fù Zǐ Xì Xīn Tāng*.
- *Má huáng* effuses and dissipates cold evil from the channels and network vessels.
- Raw *fù zǐ* warms and supplements the true yáng of shàoyīn.
- *Xì xīn* effuses the yáng qì of the kidneys and liver. The idea behind these two formulas is quite similar.
- *Má huáng* treats exterior evil; *fù zǐ* warms interior vacuity, and *xì xīn* frees evil in the yīn channels.
- However, in this formula *fù zǐ* treats exterior evil, *gān jiāng* warms interior vacuity, and *gān cǎo* harmonizes stomach yáng.
- Thus, it can be said that when raw *fù zǐ* and *gān jiāng* are combined, supplementation of the center reults in effusion, and when raw *fù zǐ* is combined with *má huáng*, effusion of the center results in supplementation.

小柴胡湯
Xiǎo Chái Hú Tāng

chái hú	柴胡	24g
huáng qín	黄芩	9g
rén shēn	人參	9g
gān cǎo	甘草	9g
bàn xià	半夏	24g
shēng jiāng	生薑	9g
dà zǎo	大棗	12 pcs

See above.

大半夏湯
Dà Bàn Xià Tāng

bàn xià	半夏	400ml
rén shēn	人參	9g
bái mì	白蜜	200ml

Indications: Treats stomach reflux and vomiting.

Analysis:

- The formula uses *bàn xià* to downbear counterflow in the thoroughfare vessel.
- Honey is used to moisten the dryness of yángmíng.
- *Rén shēn* is added to generate the already collapsed liquid and humors.
- Worked water is utilized to downbear the counterflow of water humors.
- The ingenuity lies in the use of copious amounts of water, so that the honey can be simmered for an extended period of time in order to remove the coldness of the honey and utilize its moistening function. This enables the sticky and slimy nature to remain within the stomach, and avoids the downward movement from occuring too quickly. In this way, the strength of *bàn xià* and *rén shēn* can gently mediate the center.

大黄甘草湯
Dà Huáng Gān Cǎo Tāng

dà huáng	大黄	12g
gān cǎo	甘草	6g

Indications: Treats vomiting immediately after eating, and pox sores due to phlegm oppression, which are unable to effuse outwards.

Analysis:

- When there is vomiting immediately after eating, it is suitable to use a ratio of double *dà huáng* to *gān cǎo*.
- *Dà huáng* is specifically taken to facilitate a downbearing effect in order to drain the stagnation of counterflow fullness.
- To open phlegm oppression pox sores, it is suitable to use double *dà huáng* to *gān cǎo*. This prevents the upward spilling effect of *gān cǎo*, which adversely could secure and bind the accumulation. This is a formula with few medicinals, yet its effect is extraordinary.

茯苓澤瀉湯
Fú Líng Zé Xiè Tāng

fú líng	茯苓	24g
zé xiè	澤瀉	12g
gān cǎo	甘草	6g
guì zhī	桂枝	6g
bái zhú	白朮	9g
shēng jiāng	生薑	12g

Indications: Treats stomach reflux with thirst and a desire to drink water following vomiting.

Analysis:

- In this formula, *zhū líng* is removed from *Wǔ Líng Sǎn* because there is stomach reflux with thirst, which is different than thirst following vomiting. This indicates imminent recovery.
- In a *Zhū Líng Sǎn* pattern, there is first thirst in the absence of vomiting. This is also different.
- *Shēng jiāng* and *gān cǎo* are added, and when combined with *fú líng, bái zhú* and the other medicinals are able to resolve vacuous evil in the exterior and interior, thereby harmonizing the center and stopping vomiting.

文蛤湯
Wén Gé Tāng

wén gé	文蛤	15g
shí gāo	石膏	15g
má huáng	麻黄	9g
gān cǎo	甘草	9g
shēng jiāng	生薑	9g
xìng rén	杏仁	50 kernels
dà zǎo	大棗	12 pcs

Indications: Treats thirst following vomiting with an incessant desire to drink water. This also treats mild wind with a tight pulse and headaches.

Analysis:

- Although water is expelled with vomiting, the heat is not eliminated with the water, so there is incessant, and voracious drinking of fluids.
- In the formula, *má huáng* and *shí gāo* are used together as they are able to penetrate and effuse deep-lying heat in the channels and network vessels.
- In addition, *wén gé* is used to cool and moisten the dryness, so when heat is resolved, the thirst is alleviated.
- Wind is a yáng evil, and when treating it is appropriate to cool and dissipate it. This is the reason that this formula is also able to treat it.

半夏乾薑散
Bàn Xià Gān Jiāng Sǎn

bàn xià	半夏	equal parts of each
gān jiāng	乾薑	

Indications: Treats dry retching, vomiting counterflow, and vomiting of drool and spittle.

生薑半夏湯
Shēng Jiāng Bàn Xià Tāng

bàn xià	半夏	100ml
shēng jiāng	生薑	200ml

See *Xiǎo Bàn Xià Tāng*.

橘皮湯
Jú Pí Tāng

jú pí	橘皮	12g
shēng jiāng	生薑	24g

Indications: Treats dry retching, hiccups, and reversal of the extremities.

橘皮竹茹湯
Jú Pí Zhú Rú Tāng

jú pí	橘皮	96g
zhú rú	竹茹	400ml
dà zǎo	大棗	30 pcs
shēng jiāng	生薑	24g
gān cǎo	甘草	15g
rén shēn	人參	3g

Indications: Treats stomach vacuity hiccup counterflow.

Analysis:

- Hiccup counterflow is a complex disorder resulting from the contention of cold and heat qì.
- Therefore, the formula uses *shēng jiāng* and *zhú rú*, one hot and one cold medicinal, in order to dispel the cold and heat qì, and *rén shēn* and *jú pí*, one opening and one closing medicinal in order to separate [counterflow].
- *Gān cǎo* and *dà zǎo* settle and quiet central earth, creating a powerful center earth so hiccups and counterflow are naturally calmed.

四逆湯
Sì Nì Tāng

See above.

桂枝湯
Guì Zhī Tāng

guì zhī	桂枝	9g
sháo yào	芍藥	9g
gān cǎo	甘草	6g
shēng jiāng	生薑	9g
dà zǎo	大棗	12 pcs

Indications: Treats tàiyáng disease with headache, heat effusion, sweating, aversion to wind, or mild aversion to cold, a noisy dry nose, retching, and a floating rapid pulse. These symptoms indicate disharmony of construction and defense, and thus effusing sweat is appropriate.

Analysis:

- This is Zhāng Zhòngjǐng's crowning formula to resolve the flesh, effuse sweat, and is the main formula used to harmonize the construction and defense.
- *Guì zhī* is acrid, warm, and serves to free yáng in order to treat the defense.
- *Sháo yào* is bitter, sour, and boosts yīn in order to treat the construction.
- *Shēng jiāng* is acrid, warm, and dissipates cold evil.
- *Dà zǎo* and *gān cǎo* are sweet and warm, thus supporting the central burner.
- When *guì zhī* is combined with *shēng jiāng*, the power to dispel wind and cold is increased.
- When *guì zhī* is combined with *dà zǎo*, the power of resolving the flesh and securing the exterior is increased.
- When *guì zhī* is combined with *sháo yào*, both the construction and defense are harmonized.
- When *sháo yào* is combined with *gān cǎo*, the strength of enriching and nourishing the fluids is increased.

- When the formula is taken with gruel, this assists the formulas function of promoting sweating, then the evil is eliminated without damaging liquids.
- Therefore, this formula can be used to treat all patterns of wind-cold in the exterior with a floating weak pulse, spontaneous sweating, and exterior vacuity.

大承氣湯
Dà Chéng Qì Tāng

dà huáng	大黃	12g
hòu pò	厚朴	24g
zhǐ shí	枳實	5 pcs
máng xiāo	芒硝	60ml

Indications: Repletion heat in yángmíng, with dry feces hardening and binding in the intestines, as well as fullness and pain in the abdomen.

Analysis:

- Stagnating filth in the intestines is due to qì being unable to move, and as a result fluids are unable to moisten.
- *Dà huáng* here clears heat, *máng xiāo* moistens the dryness, *hòu pò* moves the qì, and *zhǐ shí* attacks hardness.
- This formula is indicated for heat evil, which has spread to the interior manifesting with glomus, fullness, dryness, repletion, and hardness.
- If the exterior evil is not yet resolved, or there is hardness and fullness below the heart, or redness in the face, or reduced appetite, or increased retching, or a slow pulse, or internal exhaustion of the fluids causing reduced urination, any of the *Chéng Qì Tāng* formulas are contraindicated.

小承氣湯
Xiǎo Chéng Qì Tāng

dà huáng	大黃	12g
hòu pò	厚朴	6g
zhǐ shí	枳實	3 large pcs

Indications: Treats yángmíng disease with dry stool in the stomach. This also treats obstructed qì that is unable to be transported to the exterior.

Analysis:

- This formula uses *dà huáng* to control the dangerous situation as a result of extreme hyperactivity.
- The assistants' *zhǐ shí* and *hòu pò* diffuse and free stagnation in the qì aspect.
- This is a specific method used to attack accumulations.
- In *Dà Chéng Qì Tāng*, the dosage of *hòu pò* is double that of *dà huáng*, as the qì medicinal is the sovereign. *Dà Chéng Qì Tāng* is rich in flavor and fierce in nature.
- In this formula, *dà huáng* is double that of *hòu pò* as the qì medicinal is now the minister. The flavor of this formula is now scant and the nature is moderate.
- In the preparation of *Dà Chéng Qì Tāng*, first the *zhǐ shí* and *hòu pò* are boiled and *dà huáng* is added afterwards. This allows for the qì to be sharp and move easily.
- In this formula, all the medicinals are boiled together and are not cooked separately, which allows for the hardness to be attacked in such a way that it is not too harsh.

桃花湯
Táo Huā Tāng

chì shí zhī	赤石脂	48g
gān jiāng	乾薑	6g
jīng mǐ	粳米	200ml

Indications: Treats shàoyīn diarrhea with pus and blood in the stools. Additionally this treats: warm disease with a soggy and small pulse; heat removed with interior vacuity; thin and watery diarrhea with possible pus and blood in the stools.

Analysis:

- This is a method, which treats a shàoyīn pattern of direct cold strike.
- There is vacuity cold in the shàoyīn channel, which also results in vacuity cold within the intestines.
- Here, it is inappropriate to secure the blood and outwardly discharge.
- *Chì shí zhī* and *gān jiāng* are used to warm.
- *Jīng mǐ* is used to supplement.
- *Rèn shēn* can be added only if vacuity is severe.
- It is known that this is not a case of heat stagnation, therefore it is completely different than a *Bái Tóu Wēng Tāng* or a *Gé Gēn Qín Lián Tāng* pattern.

白頭翁湯
Bái Tóu Wēng Tāng

bái tóu wēng	白頭翁	6g
huáng lián	黄連	9g
huáng bǎi	黄柏	9g
qín pí	秦皮	9g

Indications: Treats juéyīn heat diarrhea with rectal heaviness, a deep and wiry pulse, and thirst with a desire to drink water.

Analysis:

- Heat diarrhea with rectal heaviness is a result of depressed fire. The steaming of dampness combined with foul qì quickly distresses the rectum and corporeal soul gate.[7] This becomes depressed and is difficult to discharge.
- This is what the *Nèi Jīng* refers to as fulminant pouring.
- The sovereign of this formula is the bitter, acrid and cold *bái tóu wēng*, which can settle the swaying of wind, calm the moving and opening of fire, while upbearing the sinking of water and qì.
- The bitter and cold astringing *qín pí* is the minister, which astringes diarrhea, and hardens efflux desertion of the liver and kidney.
- The assistant *huáng lián* clears fire in the upper burner, stopping the thirst.
- The courier *huáng bǎi* drains heat in the lower burner, and as a result diarrhea is eliminated naturally.
- Therefore, this formula is highly suitable in the initial stages of juéyīn diarrhea, however, if there is enduring diarrhea, one should use *Wū Méi Wán*.

7. Anus.

梔子豉湯
Zhī Zǐ Chǐ Tāng

zhī zǐ	梔子	14 pcs
xiāng chǐ	香豉	80ml

Indications: Opens and frees the chest and diaphragm, and treats vacuity vexation and anguish.

Analysis:

- Tàiyáng is the exterior of the heart and stomach, while yángmíng is the interior.
- Yángmíng interior is associated with stomach repletion.
- Heat effusion, aversion to heat, eye pain, dry nose, sweating, and generalized body heaviness said to be related to the exterior. Vacuity vexation, vacuity heat, dry throat, bitter taste in the mouth, the tongue coating, abdominal fullness, vexation, agitation, inability to sleep, dispersion thirst, and inhibited urination are also related to the exterior. Anything that is outside of the stomach, is related to the yángmíng exterior.
- All of Zhòngjǐng's sweating formulas open tàiyáng and offer a way out for exterior evils.
- All ejection formulas offer a method of expulsion for yángmíng exterior evils.
- Therefore in tàiyáng exterior patterns, it is appropriate to promote sweating and not to eject. Conversely, in yángmíng exterior patterns it is appropriate to eject and not to promote sweating.
- In tàiyáng disease where on the contrary ejection is used, one sees various symptoms such as spontaneous sweating, an absence of aversion to cold, hunger yet inability to eat, evening vomiting of food eaten in the morning, a desire to eat cold foods, and no desire to wear clothes. This is the result of a tàiyáng pattern shifting into the yángmíng exterior where evil heat has collected in the upper stomach duct. The method of treatment here is to administer this formula in order to eject evil.
- In the treatment of yángmíng disease where one should eject, but on the contrary effuses sweat, precipitates, or uses a warm needle, this results in symptoms such as heart fretting, fright, anguish, vexation, agitation and tongue fur. Thus, the evil is still located in the yángmíng exterior and this formula should be used.
- *Zhī zǐ* is bitter, which can eject and drain, and its coldness can overcome heat.
- *Xiāng chǐ* harmonizes the stomach and resolves the exterior. If it is stir-fried then its ability to transform turbidity and open depression is increased. When *xiāng chǐ* is combined with the bitter cold of *zhī zǐ*, these two are able to eliminate stagnant turbidity in the stomach via ejection.
- Once ejection occurs, the stomach will feel more comfortable, and vexing heat in both the exterior and interior is completely resolved.
- If one quickly eliminates stomach heat, repletion in the stomach domain is likely not eliminated.
- Therefore, this is a sacred formula to resolve the yángmíng exterior.
- If heat damages stomach qì, this results in shortness of breath. *Gān cǎo* should be added to boost the qì.
- If there is contention of vacuity and heat, this results in copious vomiting, and *shēng jiāng* should be added to stop vomiting.
- If following precipitation, there is fullness in the heart and abdomen, and disquietude whether sitting or lying, this is due to heat. In this case, the heat has already entered the

lower stomach duct, and ejection should not be used. Therefore, remove the upraising *xiāng chǐ*, and only use *zhī zǐ* to eliminate vexation, and assist *zhǐ shí* and *hòu pò* to drain fullness.

- This is a wonderful method to resolve both the heart and abdomen.
- If a pill formula is used to precipitate and generalized heat fails to leave, this signifies that the exterior has not yet resolved.
- When there is binding pain in the heart, then cold has lodged in the center. Now there is heat in the exterior and cold in the interior. Therefore to control this, use bitter *zhī zǐ* in order to eliminate heat, and use twice as much acrid *gān jiāng* in order to expel cold.
- If one provokes ejection once again by rousing stomach qì, this causes separation in the exterior. In this situation both cold and warm medicinals are used to harmonize the stomach and resolve the exterior.
- In addition, all patterns of sudden turmoil are due to stagnant dampness, which transforms into heat, and harrases the stomach. One only needs to use these two medicinals, as they are the best medicinals to address this pattern.
- If there is vomiting caused by *zhú yè*, which was used to clear summer-heat wind, then combine with *koù rén*[8] in order to diffuse foulness.
- With severe dampness use the ministers *huá shí* and *hòu pò* to overcome heat.
- When used with the assistants *fú líng* and *huáng lián*, together with *bái zhú*, *gūa dì*, and *biǎn dòu*[9] the stomach is harmonized.
- Combine with sticky *gān cǎo* in order to transform toxicity.
- If one erroneously employs warm medicinals causing agitation and derangement, this formula can also thereby rescue.
- This is indeed a major formula for the stomach domain.

通脈四逆湯
Tōng Mài Sì Nì Tāng

fù zǐ	附子	1 pc
gān jiāng	乾薑	9g
gān cǎo	甘草	6g

Indications: Treats shàoyīn disease clear food diarrhea with interior cold and exterior heat. This also treats reversal cold of the extremities with an absence of aversion to cold, a faint pulse verging on expiry, and a reddish facial complexion. There is possibly also abdominal pain, or dry retching, or throat pain, or ceasing of diarrhea where the pulse does not move outward.

Analysis:

- This formula treats exuberant yīn repelling yáng.
- When vital qì has already departed, collapse occurs quickly.
- If soft and moderate *gān cǎo* were to be used as the sovereign, one would certainly be unable to quickly dissipate yáng. Therefore, an increased dose of *gān jiāng* is used, and *gān cǎo* still does not need to be reduced.
- Thus, two aspects are covered: the return of yáng, and the preservation of fluids.

8. *Bái kòu rén* (Fructus Amomi rotundus).
9. *Bái biǎn dòu* (Semen Lablab album).

- The face is also related to the yáng vacuity upward flow, so for this reason, one can add *cōng bái* to draw yáng qì downwards.
- When there is abdominal pain due to disharmony of the spleen network vessels, remove *cōng bái* and add *sháo yào* in order to free the spleen network vessels.
- When there is retching due to upward counterflow of stomach qì, add *shēng jiāng* in order to diffuse and free.
- With throat pain associated with ascending counterflow of fire in the shàoyīn channel, remove the bitter and draining *sháo yào* and add *jié gěng* in order to open and rise.
- When diarrhea ceases, yet the pulse fails to move outwards, this is due to interior vacuity of grain qì. If the pulse fails to generate, remove the *jié gěng* and add *rén shēn* to generate the pulse.

紫參湯
Zǐ Shēn Tāng

zǐ shēn	紫參	24g
gān cǎo	甘草	9g

Indications: Treats diarrhea and lung pain.

Analysis:
- The lungs are the viscus of clearing and eliminating.
- The lungs and large intestine stand in an interior and exterior relationship, and the intestines and stomach are similarly linked together.
- Diarrhea and lung pain are due to the ascent of turbid qì from the stomach and intestines which assaults the lungs.
- *Zǐ shēn* rules the treatment of cold and heat accumulations and gatherings of evil qì in the heart and abdomen.
- *Gān cǎo* resolves the hundred toxins, and settles center earth, thus enabling the power of center earth to benefit lung metal.
- When the intestines and stomach are unobstructed, lung qì is naturally calm.
- When lung qì is calm, then its clearing and eliminating function is carried out, and the diarrhea and lung pain resolve.

訶黎勒散
Hē Lí Lè Sǎn

hē lí lè	訶黎勒	10 pcs

Indications: Treats diarrhea with loss of qì.

Analysis:
- With qì diarrhea, there is lung qì desertion.
- When both the stomach and intestines are vacuous, there is sinking qì and descent of stools.
- Quickly use *Hē Lí Lè Sǎn* to astringe the intestines and stomach in order to secure desertion.
- Also use rice gruel to support the center in order to shift qì, as once qì has shifted, diarrhea will stop on its own.

《千金翼》小承氣湯
Qiān Jīn Yì Xiǎo Chéng Qì Tāng

hòu pò	厚朴	6g
dà huáng	大黄	12g
zhǐ shí	枳實	3 pcs

Indications: Treats constipation, frequent hiccuping, and delirious speech.

《外臺》黄芩湯
Wài Tái Huáng Qín Tāng

huáng qín	黄芩	9g
rén shēn	人參	9g
gān jiāng	乾薑	9g
guì zhī	桂枝	3g
dà zǎo	大棗	12 pcs
bàn xià	半夏	100ml

Indications: Treats dry retching and diarrhea.

Analysis:

- This is Master Zhāng's variant method of *Xiǎo Chái Hú Tāng.*
- When tàiyáng disease is unresolved, it enters yángmíng, yīn and yáng are disordered, and this causes dry retching and diarrhea.
- The formula uses *huáng qín* and *gān jiāng,* one cold and one warm medicinal to advance together into the stomach in order to separate yīn and yáng.
- In addition, *bàn xià* is used to harmonize the stomach.
- *Rén shēn* and *dà zǎo* calm the stomach.
- *Guì zhī* dispels evil.
- When yīn and yáng are harmonized, then the central pivot shifts, the upper and lower interact, and the dry retching and diarrhea stop!

薏苡附子敗醬散
Yì Yǐ Fù Zǐ Bài Jiàng Sǎn

yì yǐ rén	薏苡仁	10 parts
fù zǐ	附子	2 parts
bài jiàng	敗醬	5 parts

Indications: Treats intestinal welling abscess.

Analysis:

- This is an acrid and warm formula.
- When heart qì is depressed and constrained, it binds in the head of the small intestine, obstructing the circulating path and outlet, which results in a swollen welling-abscesses.
- Just as the *Huáng Dì Nèi Jīng* says, when the viscera are unable to contain evil, the evil enters the bowels.
- Therefore, this formula uses a large dose of *yì yǐ rén* to open and free heart qì, and nourishes the region of the heart.
- The assistant *bài jiàng* transforms pus and water.
- The envoy *fù zǐ* on the one hand opens hand tàiyáng small intestine bind, and on the other transforms foot tàiyáng bladder qì. This enforces the expulsion of transformed toxicity through the waterways.

大黄牡丹湯
Dà Huáng Mǔ Dān Tāng

dà huáng	大黄	12g
mǔ dān	牡丹	3g
táo rén	桃仁	50 pcs
dōng guā rén	冬瓜仁	100ml
máng xiāo	芒硝	60ml

Indications: Treats swelling and glomus in the lesser abdomen with pain on pressure, which is similar to strangury. There is also regular urination, frequent heat effusion, spontaneous sweating, aversion to cold, and a slow and tight pulse. This indicates that pus has not yet formed.

Analysis:
- This is a pattern of welling-abscess in the large intestine.
- The formula uses a large dose of *dà huáng* and *máng xiāo* to open the large intestine bind.
- *Táo rén* and *mǔ dān* descend vanquished blood, clearing the lung, and moistening the intestines.
- Now, all that is left is *dōng guā zǐ*.
- After taking the formula there should be precipitation of blood. However, in this case, after precipitation there was no blood and only transformation of pus. By this it is known that pus has already formed, and the flesh has already decayed.
- In this case, one must first take either *Pái Nóng Sǎn* or *Tāng*.

王不留行散
Wáng Bù Liú Xíng Sǎn

wáng bù liú xíng	王不留行	10 parts
shuò diào xì yè	蒴藋細葉	10 parts
gān cǎo	甘草	18 parts
sāng dōng nán gēn	桑東南根	10 parts
huáng qín	黄芩	2 parts
shǔ jiāo	蜀椒	3 parts
hòu pò	厚朴	2 parts
gān jiāng	乾薑	2 parts
sháo yào	芍藥	2 parts

Indications: Treats incised wounds.

Analysis:
- *Wáng bù liú xíng* quickly moves the blood in the vessels and networks to irrigate the entire body, and prevents the stimulation of rushing fluids to the damaged area.
- *Sāng gēn pí* discharges wind-water from the flesh.
- *Shuò diào yè* percolates wind-water from the sinews and bones.
- These three medicinals are charred, this enables them to enter the blood, eliminate evil, and stop bleeding.
- *Chuān jiāo* dispels wind from the sore opening.
- *Hòu pò* dries the dampness in the incision.
- *Huáng lián* abates hot flesh.
- *Sháo yào* dissipates malign blood.
- *Gān jiāng* harmonizes yáng and *gān cǎo* harmonizes yīn.
- When these medicinals are used with the sovereign, they are able to enter the blood, reduce swelling, and engender flesh.
- When wind and dampness are eliminated, yīn and yáng harmonize, the sore opening disappears, and the flesh is engendered.

排膿散
Pái Nóng Sǎn

zhǐ shí	枳實	16 pcs
sháo yào	芍藥	6 parts
jié gěng	桔梗	2 parts

Indications: Treats interior welling-abscess with pus emitting from the stools.

Analysis:

- *Zhǐ shí* and *jié gěng* move qì stagnation.
- *Sháo yào* frees blood stagnation.
- Therefore, pus is eliminated through the movement of blood and qì.
- This is easy for people to understand.
- The ingenuity lies in the addition of one egg yolk, as it is an animal substance with an affinity to nourish the yīn of the heart and spleen.
- Only this method of pus expulsion can capture the root of the condition.

排膿湯
Pái Nóng Tāng

gān cǎo	甘草	6g
jié gěng	桔梗	9g
shēng jiāng	生薑	3g
dà zǎo	大棗	10 pcs

Indications: Treats interior welling-abscess with pus emitting from vomit.

Analysis:

- The formula uses acrid *jié gěng* and *shēng jiāng*, together with sweet *dà zǎo* and *gān cǎo*, as acrid and sweet medicinals are able to effuse and disperse.
- This is a yáng method, which causes toxicity to be eliminated through yáng transformation.
- This is an excellent method of expulsion.

黄連粉
Huáng Lián Fěn

Indications: Treats wet spreading sores.

Analysis:

- Wet spreading sores are an infectious disease, which can only be generated from dampness and heat.
- In order to treat them, *huáng lián's* acrid and drying nature is most appropriate.
- However, this formula has now been lost, but it is suspected that powdered *huáng lián* is the only ingredient and can either be applied externally, or ingested, and should be used accordingly.

藜蘆甘草湯
Lí Lú Gān Cǎo Tāng

Formula has been lost.

Indications: Treats patients with frequent swelling and stirring of the fingers and arms, as well as generalized twitching.

Analysis:

- Phlegm-drool is engendered from damp qì. This stagnates in the space between the chest and diaphragm, and when enduring, moves into the channel and network vessels. Therefore, numerous unpredictable changes are caused, such as frequent swelling and stirring of the fingers and arms, as well as generalized twitching.

- This is simply the result of wind-phlegm entering the network vessels.
- The nature of *lí lú* is toxic, and it is able to eject the accumulation of wind-phlegm from the chest and diaphragm.
- Once phlegm has been eliminated, then the shaking and stirring will spontaneously resolve.
- One must also consider the fact that stomach qì will be damaged following the ejection. Therefore, *gān cǎo* is used to harmonize it.

雞屎白散
Jī Shǐ Bái Sǎn

Indications: Treats cramping in the stomach.

Analysis:

- Cramping in the stomach is due to a vacuity of spleen earth, which is being exploited by liver wood.
- The chicken is a wood animal. Chicken's excrement disinhibits spleen qì, which is the reason it is able to treat this disease.
- Furthermore, since chicken feces belong to the earth class, it easily enters the spleen.

蜘蛛散
Zhī Zhū Sǎn

zhī zhū	蜘蛛	14 pcs
guì zhī	桂枝	1.5g

Indications: Treats yīn fox-like mounting qì, with testicles that change in size, and frequently ascend and descend.

Analysis:

- Yīn fox-like mounting qì is the same as the *Nèi Jīng's* fox-like mounting wind disease and this is a juéyīn channel disease.
- *Zhī zhū* has a yīn nature that is harsh. It is hidden from view and few can claim a sighting. It can calm gloomy wind, and dissipate disease in the juéyīn liver channel. With its power being in the shell, it is able to discharge bound qì in the lower burner.
- *Ròu guì* is aromatic, enters the liver, and specifically dissipates the binding of consolidated yīn that causes mounting.
- Together with *zhī zhū*, these medicinals are able to guide and abduct, making this an ingenious and divine method of treatment.

甘草粉蜜湯
Gān Cǎo Fěn Mì Tāng

gān cǎo	甘草	6g
bái fěn	白粉	3g
bái mì	白蜜	12g

Indications: Treats roundworm disease causing drooling, as well as intermittent heart pain.

Analysis:

- Within the formula *qiān fěn* is very good at killing worms.
- This is mixed with *gān cǎo* and honey, as their major sweetness can cover up *qiān fěn's* inherent toxic nature.
- This is known as first luring and then attacking.

烏梅丸
Wū Méi Wán

wū méi	烏梅	300 pcs
xì xīn	細辛	18g
gān jiāng	乾薑	30g
huáng lián	黃連	48g
dāng guī	當歸	12g
fù zǐ	附子	18g
chuān jiāo	川椒	12g
guì zhī	桂枝	18g
rén shēn	人參	18g
huáng bǎi	黃柏	18g

Indications: Treats roundworm reversal with vomiting of roundworms and enduring diarrhea.

Analysis:

- If there is enduring depression of wind-wood with failure to diffuse, then liver evil fumes and steams the stomach. The dampness and heat ferment causing the generation of roundworms.
- When there are numerous roundworms, the liver evil is boosted, therefore growing and causing reversal.
- The vomiting of roundworms emerges from the stomach and comes out through the mouth.
- This is simply a disease due to the restraining of wood and earth.
- Therefore the formula uses the majorly sour *wū méi* as the sovereign to drain the origin of the disease from the liver domain.
- The bitter and drying nature of *húang lián* and *huáng bǎi* are used as the ministers to flush out damp-heat from the stomach.
- Therefore this formula employs a strategy of using sour and bitter flavors to eject and drain, as well as to course and outthrust stagnant and depressed heat in the central burner.
- The acrid and warm *gān jiāng* and *chuān jiāo* are used as the assistants to kill the roundworms in the stomach.
- *Guì zhī*, *fù zǐ*, and *dāng guī* are the couriers, which harmonize the construction, defense, channels, and network vessels. Thus, limb reversal can also be resolved and eliminated.
- When all the medicinals are drying, acrid, and penetrating substances, there is fear of diffusing the stomach domain, thus sweet and moistening *rén shēn* is added in order to support the stomach and harmonize the other medicinals. As a result, there is no damage to the stomach qì.
- Roundworms are commonly formed from the binding of cold substances with dampness and heat.
- The sour flavor quiets roundworms, the acrid flavor subdues them, and bitterness descends them, therefore these flavors are combined along with cold and warm medicinals.
- This really is an ancestral formula for treating roundworms.
- When there is dysentery, replace the *guì zhī* with *ròu guì*, and remove the *rèn shēn*, *fù zǐ*, *xì xīn*, and *huáng bǎi*.

桂枝湯
Guì Zhī Tāng

See above.

桂枝茯苓丸
Guì Zhī Fú Líng Wán

guì zhī	桂枝	equal parts of each
fú líng	茯苓	
dān pí	丹皮	
táo rén	桃仁	
sháo yào	芍藥	

Indications: Treats women with a history of concretions.

Analysis:

- This formula uses *guì zhī* to free liver yáng.
- *Sháo yào* enriches liver yīn.
- *Fú líng* supplements heart qì.
- *Dān pí* moves heart blood.
- All is ingeniously maintained with the addition of *táo rén*, which guides all the medicinals directly into the concretion in order to attack it. This causes the stasis bind to be eliminated without damaging the new blood.

附子湯
Fù Zǐ Tāng

fù zǐ	附子	2 pcs
fú líng	茯苓	9g
rén shēn	人參	6g
bái zhú	白朮	12g
sháo yào	芍藥	9g

Indications: Treats shàoyīn disease with harmony of the mouth, cold extremities, a cold back, joint pain, and a deep pulse. This also treats painful sores due to spleen and stomach vacuity cold, or erroneous treatments involving moving, attacking or quelling, which result in reversal cold of the extremities, inability to get food down, intestinal noise, abdominal pain, retching counterflow, and vomiting. In addition it treats women in their sixth or seventh month of pregnancy with symptoms of a wiry pulse, heat effusion, increasing distension of the fetus, abdominal pain, aversion to cold, and a feeling in the lesser abdomen as if being fanned.

Analysis:

- The position of the shàoyīn channel is in the deepest portion of the body.
- When cold damage reaches this space, many cannot be saved.
- However, one can make use of *fù zǐ's* fierceness and sharpness in order to outthrust from this deep location by attacking and dissipating evil.
- Therefore the formula uses two pieces of raw *fù zǐ* as the sovereign to obtain its fierce qì. However, one must consider that *fù zǐ's* acridity and toxicity is quite severe, and can damage the post-heaven right qì. This is the reason that sweet and warm *bái zhú* is used as the minister to support it.

- The sour and sweet assistants *rén shēn* and *sháo yào* moisten post-heaven qì.
- The bland percolating *fú líng* is used as the courier to drain.
- As a result, raw *fù zǐ* can still penetrate without damaging the spleen.
- Even though raw *fù zǐ* is acrid, here it will not consume the fluids.
- Raw *fù zǐ* is toxic and drains outward, *bái zhú* banks up the earth, *sháo yào* calms wood, and *fú líng* disinhibits water. In this way when water is eliminated, fire is vigorous, and cold is naturally dispersed.
- When wood is calm, earth is boosted and secure, and water is controlled. This is mutual assistance, and as a result the cold expelling effect of raw *fù zǐ* is boosted.
- When the spleen visceral function is boosted and secured, all the various abdominal patterns are also eliminated.

膠艾湯
Jiāo Ài Tāng

gān dì huáng	乾地黃	18g
chuān xiōng	川芎	6g
ē jiāo	阿膠	6g
gān cǎo	甘草	6g
ài yè	艾葉	9g
dāng guī	當歸	9g
sháo yào	芍藥	12g

Indications: Treats abdominal pain with spotting in pregnancy due to uterine obstruction. This also treats blood descent or incessant bleeding following late miscarriage.

Analysis:

- *Chuān xiōng, sháo yào*, and *dì huáng* are blood-supplementing medicinals.
- Blood is not generated on its own, but is engendered from water and grains in yángmíng, therefore *gān cǎo* is used to supplement yángmíng.
- *Ē jiāo* enriches the sea of blood, and is a very important medicinal for treating various pregnancy related diseases.
- *Ài yè* warms the uterus, and is a specific medicinal to regulate menstruation and calm the fetus.
- This is a divine formula, which unites juéyīn, shàoyīn and yángmíng, while simultaneously treating the thoroughfare and controlling vessels.

當歸芍藥散
Dāng Guī Sháo Yào Sǎn

dāng guī	當歸	9g
chuān xiōng	川芎	9g
sháo yào	芍藥	48g
fú líng	茯苓	12g
bái zhú	白朮	12g
zé xiè	澤瀉	24g

Indications: Treats dull abdominal pain in pregnant women, urgent pain below the heart, postpartum blood dizziness, vacuity of the eyes, a lack of qì, flooding, and enduring diarrhea. Taking this formula for an extended period of time frees and disinhibits the vessels, dispels phlegm, nourishes the kidneys, brightens the eyes, boosts liquids, dispels wind, supplements taxation, nourishes true yáng, abates evil heat, harmonizes the spirit, moistens and enriches the face, dissipates cold evil, and warms miasmic qì.

Analysis:

- Abdominal pain in pregnancy is commonly associated with congealed blood and qì depression, therefore *dāng guì* and *sháo yào* are used to dissipate them.
- Because the liver is the sea of blood, this method fulfills the liver's desire to be uninhibited and outthrust.
- Blood is engendered by center qì. The center is earth. When there is excessive dryness of the earth, it is unable to generate anything, so for this reason the enriching medicinals *dāng guī, chuān xiōng* and *sháo yào* are used.
- Excess dampness in the earth is also unable to generate anything, so *fú líng, bái zhú,* and *zé xiè* are used to percolate it.
- When dryness and dampness are appropriately addressed, center qì will be at peace, blood will be engendered on its own, and pain will cease.

乾薑人參半夏丸
Gān Jiāng Rén Shēn Bàn Xià Wán

gān jiāng	乾薑	3g
rén shēn	人參	3g
bàn xià	半夏	6g

Indications: Treats incessant vomiting in pregnancy.

當歸貝母苦參丸
Dāng Guī Bèi Mǔ Kǔ Shēn Wán

dāng guī	當歸	12g
bèi mǔ	貝母	12g
kǔ shēn	苦參	12g

Indications: Treats difficult urination with normal eating and drinking in pregnancy.

Analysis:

- This pattern is caused by depressed heat and drying of the fluids.
- Therefore, *kǔ shēn* and *dāng guī* are used to supplement heart blood and clear heart fire.
- *Bèi mǔ* opens lung depression and drains lung fire.
- When heart fire descends, then there is an absence of short rough voidings of urine and lung qì moves. As a result, the waterways of the bladder are free.
- This formula utilizes the method of addressing the upper to treat disease in the lower body.

葵子茯苓散
Kuí Zǐ Fú Líng Sǎn

kuí zǐ	葵子	200ml
fú líng	茯苓	9g

Indications: Treats water qì in pregnancy, with generalized heaviness, inhibited urination, aversion to cold as after soaking, and dizziness on rising.

當歸散
Dāng Guī Sǎn

dāng guī	當歸	48g
huáng qín	黄芩	48g
sháo yào	芍藥	48g
chuān xiōng	川芎	48g
bái zhú	白朮	24g

Indications: Clears heat, calms the fetus, and thus it is suitable to be taken frequently throughout pregnancy. This also treats several postpartum diseases.

Analysis:

- The large and small intestines are coiled and bound within the abdomen. There are numerous blood vessels assembled in front of the intestines.
- During pregnancy, there is equal pressure on both the vessels and intestines. This causes stoppage and stagnation, which results in the generation of heat.
- Therefore, the formula uses *bái zhú* to fortify the intestines.
- *Huáng qín* clears heat in the intestines.
- *Dāng guī* and *chuān xiōng* move stagnation in the blood vessels.
- *Sháo yào* drains heat in the blood vessels.

白朮散
Bái Zhú Sǎn

bái zhú	白朮	3 parts
chuān xiōng	川芎	3 parts
shǔ jiāo	蜀椒	3 parts
mǔ lì	牡蠣	no amount given

Indications: Treats fetal cold and vaginal discharge.

Analysis:

- In earlier versions of the book, this formula used three parts each of the first three ingredients, while the dosage of ***mǔ lì*** was missing.
- However, according to the formulas method of administration of three doses per day, and one dose at night, using one part ***mǔ lì*** is acceptable.

小柴胡湯
Xiǎo Chái Hú Tāng

See above.

大承氣湯
Dà Chéng Qì Tāng

See above.

當歸生薑羊肉湯
Dāng Guī Shēng Jiāng Yáng Ròu Tāng

dāng guī	當歸	9g
shēng jiāng	生薑	15g
yáng ròu	羊肉	48g

Indications: Treats cold mounting abdominal pain, vacuity taxation and insufficiency, and incessant postpartum abdominal pain.

Analysis:

- The formula uses *dāng guī* to settle pain by moving stagnation in the blood aspect.
- *Shēng jiāng* settles pain by diffusing stagnation in the qì aspect.
- *Yáng ròu* (mutton) is a substance with an affinity for qì and blood; its qì and flavor are rank and thick, and it is able to enrich and supplement.
- Cold mounting should be attacked with warmth, but in patients with vacuity taxation and insufficiency, one should not attack.
- Abdominal pain should be treated by freeing and discharging. However, in postpartum vacuity patterns, one should not discharge.
- Therefore, this method here is designed to both free and supplement. As a result blood is moved without being damaged; qì is disinhibited without being consumed; and once both qì and blood are free and disinhibited, pain will resolve on its own.

枳實芍藥散
Zhǐ Shí Sháo Yào Sǎn

zhǐ shí	枳實	equal parts
sháo yào	芍藥	equal parts

Indications: Treats postpartum abdominal pain, vexation, fullness, and sleeplessness.

Analysis:

- *Zhǐ shí* frees qì stagnation, while *sháo yào* frees blood stagnation.
- Free flow results in the absence of pain, which is common knowledge amongst the people.
- The ingenuity of this formula lies in charring *zhǐ shí*, which when transformed by fire, is excellent at attacking collections and accumulations.
- When the formula is taken with barley gruel, the liver qì is harmonized, while the heart and spleen are simultaneously nourished.
- The intention of this formula is to move stagnation, while supplementing and nourishing. This is the reason it also rules the treatment of welling-abscesses with pus.

下瘀血湯
Xià Yū Xuè Tāng

dà huáng	大黃	9g
táo rén	桃仁	20 pcs
zhè chóng	蟅蟲	20 pcs

Indications: Treats postpartum abdominal pain due to static blood below the umbilicus. It also rules the treatment of inhibited menstruation.

Analysis:

- In this formula *dà huáng* and *táo rén* are used to push out the old by precipitating stasis.
- *Zhè chóng* attacks dry blood.
- When combined with *táo rén*, these two medicinals directly enter the blood aspect to both harmonize and dissipate, there by expelling the old, while not damaging the new.

大承氣湯
Dà Chéng Qì Tāng

See above.

陽旦湯
Yáng Dàn Tāng

Guì Zhī Tāng with double *guì zhī* and the addition of *fù zǐ*.

Indications: Treats postpartum wind strike, which remains unresolved for several tens of days with a mild headache, aversion to cold, frequent heat effusion, oppression below the heart, dry retching, and sweating.

Analysis:

- Headaches, heat effusion, aversion to cold, and sweating are symptoms associated with a tàiyáng exterior pattern.
- When there is oppression below the heart, tàiyáng water evil has pervaded the area below the heart and causes oppression.
- Although there is a lack of resolution ten days postpartum, the evil is still located in the tàiyáng channel, and it is for this reason that *Guì Zhī Tāng* is used to resolve exterior evil in the tàiyáng.
- *Guì zhī* is increased in order to transform water qì in the bladder.
- *Fù zǐ* is added to the formula to warm and secure the water viscus, enabling the transformation of qì in the channels and viscera, and ensuring the expulsion of evils in both the interior and exterior.

竹葉湯
Zhú Yè Tāng

zhú yè	竹葉	one handful
gé gēn	葛根	9g
fáng fēng	防風	3g
jié gěng	桔梗	3g
guì zhī	桂枝	3g
rén shēn	人參	3g
gān cǎo	甘草	3g
fù zǐ	附子	1 pc
shēng jiāng	生薑	15g
dà zǎo	大棗	15 pcs

Indications: Treats postpartum wind strike, heat effusion, a full red facial complexion, panting and headaches.

Analysis:

- A condition that has not yet become as severe as arched-back rigidity, but that has heat effusion, a red facial complexion, and headaches. This is the beginning of wind tetany.
- Therefore, *zhú yè* is used, as it rules wind tetany. *Fáng fēng* treats internal tetany, *gé gēn* treats hard tetany, and *guì zhī* treats soft tetany.

- *Shēng jiāng* dissipates wind evil, while *jié gěng* eliminates wind impediment.
- This prescription utilizes acrid medicinals in order to dissipate.
- In addition, these are assisted by *rén shēn*, which engenders fluids to nourish the sinews, and *fù zǐ*, which moves the channels to supplement fire.
- These are all combined with *gān cǎo*, which harmonizes all the medicinals, and *dà zǎo*, which assists all twelve channels.
- All together this is a wind prescription, which contains ingredients to effuse, dissipate, and at the same time supplement, making it the most suitable prescription for postpartum wind strike.

竹皮大丸
Zhú Pí Dà Wán

zhú rú	竹茹	2 parts
shí gāo	石膏	2 parts
guì zhī	桂枝	1 part
bái wēi	白薇	1 part
gān cǎo	甘草	7 parts

Indications: Calms the center and boosts qì in order to treat vacuity in women during lactation, who also have vexing confusion and retching counterflow.

Analysis:

- When there is vacuity in lactation, it is said that the excessive suckling of milk by the child results in vacuity.
- When there is vacuity of the center, blood is unable to nourish the heart resulting in vexation, and when there is disquietude of the heart spirit, there is confusion.
- When yáng qì ascends, this results in retching.
- With counterflow, the retching is severe.
- The formula uses *zhú rú* to downbear counterflow and stop vomiting.
- *Bái wēi* eliminates heat and abates vexation.
- *Shí gāo* frees milk and settles confusion.
- A large dose of *gān cǎo* is used with *dà zǎo* to stabilize and calm the central burner in order to engender fluids.
- Blood is unable to move without yáng qì, which is why *guì zhī* is ingeniously added to move qì and blood, revere the heart, and free the milk.
- As a result, the retching counterflow will stop, the center will immediately be calmed on its own, vexing confusion will be abated, and qì will be boosted naturally.

白頭翁加甘草阿膠湯
Bái Tóu Wēng Jiā Gān Cǎo Ē Jiāo Tang

bái tóu wēng	白頭翁	6g
ē jiāo	阿膠	6g
gān cǎo	甘草	6g
huáng lián	黃連	9g
huáng bǎi	黃柏	9g
qín pí	秦皮	9g

Indications: Treats heat diarrhea with pus and blood. This also treats postpartum diarrhea and extreme vacuity.

Analysis:

- Postpartum excessive blood loss, and simultaneous diarrhea will result in collapse of fluids.

- It can be said that in extreme vacuity one should rectify with major supplementation, yet if medicinals such as *dāng guī, chuān xiōng, sháo yào,* and *dì huáng* are used they can increase the efflux and cause downward desertion.
- If *rén shēn, bái zhú, guì zhī,* and *huáng qí* are used, they can stir yáng and cause ascending counterflow.
- One needs only to use the major bitterness of *Bái Tóu Wēng Tāng* in order to rescue yīn and drain heat in the blood aspect.
- In addition, sweet *gān cǎo* is used to harmonize and regulate, and thus a method to form yīn using bitter and sweet medicinals is utilized.
- Moreover, frequent pus and blood in the stools, and diarrhea will result in desertion.
- Give enriching and moistening *ē jiāo* in combination with *Bái Tóu Wēng Tāng* to effectively harden the yīn, thus both the source and development of the condition are cleared, and the diarrhea will stop on its own.

《千金》三物黄芩湯
Qiān Jīn Sān Wù Huáng Qín Tāng

huáng qín	黄芩	3g
kǔ shēn	苦參	6g
gān dì huáng	乾地黄	12g

Indications: Treats postpartum muddledness and wind. If there is heat in the extremities and headache, give *Xiǎo Chái Hú Tāng*. If there are no headaches and only vexation give this formula.

Analysis:

- When women have just given birth their blood is vacuous.
- Juéyīn rules the blood. When blood is vacuous, juéyīn ministerial fire stirs, and when this fire stirs, the pores open. Thus, wind evil exploits the vacuity and attacks.
- *Xiǎo Chái Hú Tāng* is given to outthrust evil, which allows the evil to be expelled outwards from the pivot.
- If there are no headaches, and only vexation, wind evil is depressed internally and agitates the heat within the pericardium. When pericardium heat is intense, blood is damaged, and therefore these indications are ruled by this formula.
- *Dì huáng* is used, as it is sweet and cold with abundant thick fluids, which then supplement the vacuity of both yīn and blood.
- *Huáng qín* is bitter and cold, which can drain heat in the pericardium, allowing for the pacifying of fire, and extinguishing of wind.
- When yīn is restored, and the liver is peaceful, then the vexing heat in the four extremities spontaneously resolves.
- Moreover, when there is heat in the pericardium this is complicated by wind wood, which engenders worms. This is the reason why after taking the formula there may be profuse vomiting or precipitation of worms.

《千金》內補當歸建中湯
Qiān Jīn Nèi Bǔ Dāng Guī Jiàn Zhōng Tāng

dāng guī	當歸	12g
guì zhī	桂枝	9g
sháo yào	芍藥	18g
shēng jiāng	生薑	9g
gān cǎo	甘草	6g
dà zǎo	大棗	12 pcs

Indications: Treats postpartum vacuity emaciation; insufficiency with incessant stabbing pain in the center of the abdomen; and shortage of qì despite heavy inhalations. There may also possibly be hypertonicity and pain in the lesser abdomen stretching to the lower back and back, and an inability to eat or drink.

Analysis:

- Postpartum shortage of qì despite heavy inhalations with an inability to eat and drink, means that the disease is in tàiyīn.
- Incessant stabbing pain in the abdomen or hypertonicity and pain in the lesser abdomen stretching to the lower back and back, means the disease is in juéyīn.
- When the disease belongs to vacuity emaciation and insufficiency *Guì Zhī Tāng* with double *sháo yào* is used in order to assist the weakness of spleen qì.
- Pulling and stabbing pain are due to blood stasis, therefore, *dāng guī* is used in order to free the congealing and gathering of stasis, giving spleen qì the power to transport upwards and turn downwards.
- Taken frequently over the first month after giving birth will provide women with strength, as it has a supplementing and boosting effect.
- As for the addition of *yí táng*, when there is major vacuity of center earth a sowing and reaping flavor is used in order to supplement the qì and blood of the central burner.
- If there is excessive blood loss, flooding, or incessant spontaneous internal bleeding, this means that the sea of blood is empty and vacuous, and further, yīn qì fails to keep to its abode. Thus *dì huáng* and *ē jiāo's* heavy turbidity and thick flavor are added to nourish yin.
- The name of the formula means to supplement the interior, for postpartum vacuity emaciation, is primarily a disease of the interior.

小柴胡湯
Xiǎo Chái Hú Tāng

See above.

半夏厚朴湯
Bàn Xià Hoù Pò Tāng

bàn xià	半夏	200ml
hòu pò	厚朴	9g
fú líng	茯苓	12g
shēng jiāng	生薑	15g
sū yè	蘇葉	6g

Indications: Treats women who feel as if there is a piece of fried meat in their throat. Also treats glomus and fullness in the stomach duct, nausea, and retching counterflow. The onset of all depression patterns is due to cold and repletion.

Analysis:

- In this formula *bàn xià* downbears counterflow qì.
- *Hòu pò* resolves bound qì.
- *Fú líng* disperses phlegm.
- The particularly ingenious *shēng jiāng* is used to promote the enlightenment of the spirit, while assisting the right qì in expelling evils.
- The acrid and fragrant *sū yè* dissipates depressed qì.
- Once the depression is dissipated, and qì is regulated, the congealed and bound phlegm are transformed.
- In later times, people constructed and modeled the formula *Qī Qì Tāng* around this formula.

甘麥大棗湯
Gān Mài Dà Zǎo Tāng

gān cǎo	甘草	9g
xiǎo mài	小麥	200ml
dà zǎo	大棗	10 pcs

Indications: Treats visceral agitation in women with a tendancy to sorrow.

小青龍湯
Xiǎo Qīng Lóng Tāng

má huáng	麻黄	18g
guì zhī	桂枝	9g
gān cǎo	甘草	6g
xìng rén	杏仁	14 pcs
shēng jiāng	生薑	9g
dà zǎo	大棗	12 pcs
shí gāo	石膏	size of a large egg

See above.

瀉心湯
Xiè Xīn Tāng

dà huáng	大黃	6g
huáng lián	黃連	3g
huáng qín	黃芩	3g

See above.

溫經湯
Wēn Jīng Tāng

wú zhū yú	吳茱萸	9g
dāng guī	當歸	6g
xiōng qióng	芎藭	6g
sháo yào	芍藥	6g
rén shēn	人參	6g
guì zhī	桂枝	6g
ē jiāo	阿膠	6g
dān pí	丹皮	6g
gān cǎo	甘草	6g
shēng jiāng	生薑	9g

bàn xià	半夏	100ml
mài dōng	麥冬	200ml

Indications: Treats women in their fifties who suffer from incessant diarrhea more than ten times per day, with heat effusion in the evening, lesser abdominal urgency, abdominal fullness, vexing heat in the palms, and dry lips and mouth. This also treats adverse menstrual flow and vacuity cold inferitility.

Analysis:

- This is an ancestral formula used to regulate the menses.
- *Mài dōng* enriches stomach fluids.
- *Rén shēn* supplements stomach qì.
- *Shēng jiāng* moves stomach qì.
- *Bàn xià* harmonizes stomach qì, as once stomach qì is normalized, then the essence of water and grains can be digested much easier.
- When yáng arises, yīn grows, and thus blood can be full.
- *Ē jiāo* supplements the insufficiency of blood, while the sour and sweet flavor of *sháo yào* and *gān cǎo* are used to assist it.
- *Dāng guī* and *chuān xiōng* move the stoppage and stagnation of blood.
- *Dān pí* eliminates latent fire from the blood.
- *Guì zhī* is used to harmonize the nutritive and defense.
- *Wú zhū yú* harmonizes the liver and stomach.
- This formula attaches great importance to yángmíng, which is signified by using cold, warm, enriching and drying medicinals without emphasis on any particular one.
- Therefore it is able to control and treat the thirty-six women's diseases.
- If the menses are scanty it can free it, and if there is copious menstruation it can stop it.
- When there is vacuity cold of the uterus, it can make one pregnant.
- None of the later generation of formulas used to regulate the menses even come close to the scope of this formula.

土瓜根散
Tǔ Guā Gēn Sǎn

tǔ guā gēn	土瓜根	3 parts
sháo yào	芍藥	3 parts
guì zhī	桂枝	3 parts
zhè chóng	蟅蟲	3 parts

Indications: Treats women's diseases with inhibited menstruation, fullness and pain in the lesser abdomen, and menses that appear twice a month.

Analysis:

- This formula harmonizes yīn and yáng, expels heat, and frees stasis.
- The formula uses *guì zhī* to free yáng, and *sháo yào* to move yīn, bringing forth the harmony of yīn and yáng, which results in the regulation of the foundation of the menses.
- *Tǔ guā gēn* expels heat and moves stasis.
- *Zhè chóng* causes peristalsis in order to move the blood, thus expelling the old to engender the new.
- As a result the menses is naturally uninhibited.

旋覆花湯
Xuán Fù Huā Tāng

xuán fù huā	旋覆花	9g
cōng	葱	14 stems
xīn jiàng	新絳	small amount

See above.

膠薑湯
Jiāo Jiāng Tāng

Indications: Treats women with fallen menstruation manifesting with incessant spotting of dark blood.

Analysis:

- This formula has been lost. Some claim that this formula is simply just *gān jiāng* and *ē jiāo* taken together as a decoction, while others claim it is *Jiāo Ài Tāng.*
- This formula is most likely *Jiāo Jiāng Tāng* with just the two medicinals *shēng jiāng* and *ē jiāo.*
- *Ē jiāo* nourishes the blood, calms the liver, eliminates stasis, and engenders the new.
- *Shēng jiāng* dissipates cold and ascends qì, thus lifting what is sinking.
- Therefore the meaning behind the formula is to dissipate depression, supplement damage, and to nourish.

大黃甘遂湯
Dà Huáng Gān Suì Tāng

dà huáng	大黃	12g
gān suì	甘遂	6g
ē jiāo	阿膠	6g

Indications: Treats women with lower abdominal fullness that resembles a *duì,* with slight difficulty in urination, and an absence of thirst.

Analysis:

- This pattern is due to the binding of both water and blood in the blood chamber.
- Within the formula *dà huáng* attacks the blood amassment.
- *Gān suì* attacks the water amassment.
- *Ē jiāo* is used to save the source of water and harmonize the blood.
- This excellent method eliminates the amassment of both water and blood.

抵當湯
Dǐ Dàng Tāng

shuǐ zhì	水蛭	20 pcs
méng chóng	虻蟲	30 pcs
táo rén	桃仁	20 pcs
dà huáng	大黃	9g

Indications: Treats blood amassment due to cold damage with mania, forgetfulness, hardness and fullness in the lower abdomen, spontaneously uninhibited urination, dark colored stools, generalized yellowing, and a deep and bound pulse. This also treats women with inhibited menstruation and a repletion pulse.

Analysis:

- In tàiyáng there is a distinction between the channels and the qì, as well as a differentiation between the outer body and the exterior.
- A *Táo Rén Chéng Qì Tāng* pattern consists of heat binding in the bladder, as well as the lodging of evil in the tàiyáng fleshy exterior. Evil descends from the back and paravertebral sinews down into the bladder, which is why it is said that the outer body is unresolved, and one cannot attack.
- The fleshy exterior is the outer body.
- A *Dǐ Dàng Tāng* pattern is the result of static heat in the interior and evil in the tàiyáng exterior skin. Evil descends down from the chest, and binds in the lower abdomen. Exterior qì passes through the chest, as tàiyáng rules this cycle of qì.
- However, the exterior pattern is still present.
- The pulse should be floating when there is interior binding in the chest. Now, on the contrary, there is no binding in the chest, and the pulse is faint and deep. From this we know that exterior evil has descended from the chest and entered the yīn aspect.
- Yīn is unable to overcome yáng and therefore, there is mania.
- When heat is in the lower burner, there is hard fullness in the lower abdomen.
- When there is hardness and fullness with spontaneously uninhibited urination, we also know that evil is not present in the formless qì aspect, but is present in the formed blood aspect.
- This formula uses *méng chóng* and *shuǐ zhì*, one substance that flies, and another that stealthily sucks the blood.
- When there is heat that follows the channels and enters the upper body, the flying substance is able to reach it.
- When there is heat in the blood of the lower body that is static, the stealth substance should be used.
- They are combined with *táo hé*, to supply impressive strength to the troops, which can descend to beat and resist the major enemy.
- These four medicinals are appropriate to treat this pattern, and are thus the reason this formula is referred to as the resistance decoction.
- This formula is also suitable for women with inhibited menstruation, whose pulse and pattern are both replete. Otherwise in the absence of repletion, one should nourish the source of the thoroughfare and conception vessels, and not offensively precipitate.

礬石丸
Fán Shí Wán

fán shí	礬石	3 parts
xìng rén	杏仁	1 part

Indications: Treats women with blocked or inhibited menstruation, incessant hard aggregation in the uterus with dry blood inside, and discharge of a white substance.

Analysis:

- When there is incessant hard aggregation with dry blood in the uterus, this is due to hardness that has accumulated and become an aggregation, which fails to leave.

- Dry blood is not eliminated, thus new blood is unable to flourish, and therefore menstruation becomes blocked or inhibited.
- Due to the periodic discharging of the amassment, the uterus generates dampness, which in turn engenders heat. The place where the damp-heat accumulates is in the blood. The dry blood is corroded by the dampness and heat, and becomes a white substance, which then frequently discharges.
- Here it is appropriate to first eliminate the visceral uterine dampness and heat.
- *Fán shí* eliminates both water and heat, and when combined with *xìng rén*, is able to break bind and moisten the dry blood. Therefore, this formula rules the treatment of this pattern.

紅藍花酒
Hóng Lán Huā Jiǔ

hóng lán huā	紅藍花	3g

Indications: Treats the sixty-two kinds of wind in women with blood and qì stabbing pain in the abdomen, as well as malaria.

Analysis:
- Wind diseases in women are typically the result of blood vacuity, therefore, ***hóng huā*** is used in order to engender and move blood.
- Wine has the ability to affect the defensive qì by first moving in the skin. Therefore, by simmering the medicinal in wine, it's nature is assisted.
- This also treats malaria, as this condition is caused by malaria evil. The malaria evil hides between the interstices and the membrane source, thus this formula is able to outwardly expel this evil.

當歸芍藥散
Dāng Guī Sháo Yào Săn

dāng guī	當歸	9g
sháo yào	芍藥	24g
fú líng	茯苓	12g
bái zhú	白朮	12g
zé xiè	澤瀉	24g
chuān xiōng	川芎	24g

See above.

小建中湯
Xiǎo Jiàn Zhōng Tāng

guì zhī	桂枝	9g
gān cǎo	甘草	9g
dà zǎo	大棗	12 pcs
sháo yào	芍藥	18g
shēng jiāng	生薑	9g
jiāo yí	膠飴	200ml

See above.

腎氣丸
Shèn Qì Wán

gān dì huáng	乾地黃	24g
shān yào	山藥	12g
shān zhū yú	山茱萸	12g
fú líng	茯苓	9g
dān pí	丹皮	9g
zé xiè	澤瀉	9g
fù zǐ	附子	1 pc
guì zhī	桂枝	3g

See above.

蛇床子散
Shé Chuáng Zǐ Sǎn

shé chuáng zǐ 蛇床子

Indications: Treats genital cold in women.

狼牙湯
Láng Yá Tāng

láng yá 狼牙 9g

Indications: A treatment for sores, which have putrified and caused damage to the vagina. These sores manifest themselves with dripping pus and a foul smell.

Indices

Texts

People

Medicinals

Formulas

金匱方歌括

Indications

D

H

I

M

N

O

P

T

W

Y

The Chinese Medicine Database

www.cm-db.com

The Chinese Medicine Database has been organized around one central principle -- translation of Classical Chinese texts, and dissemination of that information.

There are thousands of Chinese medicine texts that have never been translated. We have compiled a small list on our website of the ones that we have found, but we believe that there are tens of thousands of documents that span from the *Hàn* Dynasty to pre-Republican times. Most of these documents will never be read by people in the West, simply because of lack of translation.

We have created a vehicle, that allows interested practitioners, students, institutions, and scholars to help support and fund the translation of these documents, and then mine and synthesize the data that is gained from these texts.

The Database contains:

Monographs on:

690 Single Herbs
1510 Formulas
Mayway's Patents
ITM's Formulations
Golden Flowers Formulations
Classical Pearls Formulations by Heiner Fruehauf
OBGYN Modifications to Formulas
Single Points: the 361 Regular Points
Time Line of the History of Chinese Medicine

Beer Hall Lecture Series

Watch videos from our monthly Beer Hall lecture series with guest speakers such as: Arnaud Versluys, Subhuti Dharmananda, Jason Robertson, Craig Mitchell, Michael Max, Lorraine Wilcox, and Ed Neal.

Play STORT

Play our free online game STORT where you can learn Chinese while having a bit of fun (www.cm-db.com/stort).

15,000 Western Diagnoses with ICD-9 Codes

A Chinese-English dictionary:

Containing over 102,271 terms, including the Eastland and the WHO term sets.

A Western Book search containing:

Fenner's Complete Formulary
by B. Fenner

The 1918 Dispensatory of the United States of America
Edited by Joseph P. Remington, Horatio C. Woods and others
The Eclectic Materia Medica, Pharmacology and Therapeutics
by Harvey Wickes Felter, M.D.

A Personal Dashboard, which allows users to:

Blog
Take notes on any monograph.
Search for other users by city, state, country and name.
Make friends all around the world.
Share and compare notes with friends.
Personalize your dashboard by adding photos, and information about your practice.

Translations:

Shāng Hán Lái Sū Jí	傷寒來蘇集	Renewal of Treatise on Cold Damage
Qí Jīng Bā Mài Kǎo	奇經八脈考	Explanation of the Eight Vessels of the Marvellous Meridians
Shāng Hán Míng Lǐ Lùn	傷寒明理論	Treatise on Enlightening the Principles of Cold Damage
Wú Jū Tōng Yī Àn	吴鞠通医案	Case Studies of Wú Jūtōng
The Nàn Jīng	難經	The Classic of Difficulties
The Zàng Fǔ Biāo Běn Hán Rè Xū Shí Yòng Yào Shì	臟腑標本寒熱虛實用藥式	Viscera and Bowels, Tip and Root, Cold and Heat, Vacuity and Repletion Model for Using Medicinals
Wēn Rè Lún	温熱論	Treatise on Warm Heat Disease
Shāng Hán Shé Jiàn	傷寒舌鑒	Tongue Mirror of Cold Damage
Xǔ Shì Yī Àn	許氏醫案	Case Histories of Master Xǔ
Fǔ Xìng Jué Zāng Fǔ Yòng Yào Fǎ Yào	輔行决臟腑用藥法要	Secret Instructions for Assisting the Body: Essential Methods for the Application of Drugs to the Viscera & Bowels
Biāo Yōu Fù	標幽賦	Indicating the Obscure
Liú Juān Zǐ Guǐ Yí Fāng	劉涓子鬼遺方	Liu Juanzi's Formulas Inherited from Ghosts
Shèn Jí Chú Yán	慎疾芻言	Precautions in Illness: My Humble Thoughts
Yào Zhèng Jì Yí	藥症忌宜	Medicinals & Patterns Contraindications & Appropriate [Choices]
Fù Kē Wèn Dá	婦科問答	Questions and Answers in Gynecology
Nèi Jīng Zhī Yào	內經知要	Essential Knowledge from the Nèijīng

Benefits:

Subscribers to the Database receive a 10% discount on our published books when they are in pre-release.

We translate texts as often, and in quantities that reflect our user base. The larger amount of subscribers that we have, the more translation that we can accomplish.

Published Books:

2008 Bèi Jí Qiān Jīn Yào Fāng 備急千金要方: Essential Prescriptions Worth a Thousand Gold Pieces For Emergencies. vol. 2-4 by Sūn Sīmiǎo 孫思邈
Translated by Sabine Wilms.
ISBN 978-0-9799552-0-4

2010 Zhēn Jiǔ Dà Chéng 針灸大成: The Great Compendium of Acupuncture & Moxabustion vol. I by Yáng Jìzhōu 楊繼洲
Translated by Sabine Wilms.
ISBN 978-0-9799552-2-8

2010 Zhēn Jiǔ Dà Chéng 針灸大成: The Great Compendium of Acupuncture & Moxabustion vol. V by Yáng Jìzhōu 楊繼洲
Translated by Lorraine Wilcox.
ISBN 978-0-9799552-4-2

2010 Jīn Guì Fāng Gē Kuò 金匱方歌括: Formulas from the Golden Cabinet with Songs vol. I - III by Chén Xiūyuán 陳修園
Translated by Sabine Wilms.
ISBN 978-0-9799552-5-9

2011 Zhēn Jiǔ Dà Chéng 針灸大成: The Great Compendium of Acupuncture & Moxabustion vol. VIII by Yáng Jìzhōu 楊繼洲
Translated by Yue Lu.
ISBN 978-0-9799552-7-3

2011 Zhēn Jiǔ Dà Chéng 針灸大成: The Great Compendium of Acupuncture & Moxabustion vol. IX by Yáng Jìzhōu 楊繼洲
Translated by Lorraine Wilcox.
ISBN 978-0-9799552-6-6

2012 Raising the Dead and Returning Life: Emergency Medicine of the Qīng Dynasty by Bào Xiāng'áo 鮑相璈
Translated by Lorraine Wilcox.
ISBN 978-0-9799552-3-5

2014 Zhēn Jiǔ Zī Shēng Jīng 針灸資生經: The Classic of Supporting Life with Acupuncture and Moxibustion Vol. I-III by Wáng Zhízhōng 王執中
Translated by Yue Lu.
ISBN 978-0-9799552-1-1

www.ingramcontent.com/pod-product-compliance
Lightning Source LLC
LaVergne TN
LVHW082346011026
849160LV00024B/1184
* 9 7 8 0 9 7 9 9 5 5 2 8 0 *